AIDS: Safety, Sexuality and Risk

Social Aspects of AIDS
Series Editor: Peter Aggleton
Institute of Education, University of London

Editorial Advisory Board

AIDS:
Safety, Sexuality and Risk

Edited by
Peter Aggleton, Peter Davies and Graham Hart

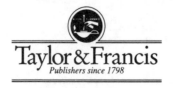

Taylor & Francis
Publishers since 1798

| UK | Taylor & Francis Ltd, 4 John St., London WC1N 2ET |
| USA | Taylor & Francis Inc., 1900 Frost Road, Suite 101, Bristol, PA 19007 |

First published 1995

A Catalogue Record for this book is available from the British Library

ISBN 0 7484 0291 8
ISBN 0 7484 0292 6 pbk

**Library of Congress Cataloging-in-Publication Data are available
on request**

Series cover design by Barking Dog Art

Typeset in 10/12 pt Baskerville
by Solidus (Bristol) Limited

Printed in Great Britain by SRP Ltd., Exeter

Contents

Contents

Preface

Some 12 years into the epidemic, and with an effective preventive vaccine or therapy against HIV disease still to be found, it is appropriate to reflect on the contribution of social and behavioural research to the development of interventions for prevention. After over a decade's work documenting HIV and AIDS-related knowledge, attitudes and behaviour, social researchers have begun to focus more closely on perceptions of sexual and drug-related safety and risk, the factors that contribute to these, and the role of non-governmental and community-based organizations in facilitating accurate risk assessment.

These issues were examined during three major conferences in 1994: the annual conference of the British Sociological Association, the 2nd International Conference on the BioPsycho-Social Aspects of AIDS, and the Xth International Conference on AIDS. This book brings together key papers presented at each of these conferences, documenting issues of focal concern to social researchers, policy makers and health educators in the mid-1990s.

In addition to all who participated in these meetings, and who revised the presentations they gave for inclusion in this book, we would like to thank Helen Thomas for preparing the final manuscript for publication.

Peter Aggleton
Peter Davies
Graham Hart

Chapter 1

Reputedly Effective Risk Reduction Strategies and Gay Men

Marie-Ange Schiltz and Philippe Adam

The outbreak of AIDS has overwhelmed the entire gay world. The initial drop in the frequency of 'casual' sexual encounters, first observed in France in our second study in 1986 (Pollak and Schiltz, 1987), has been followed by the development of various strategies that enable gay men to continue to have this kind of sexual activity. Although the prevention message directed at gay men in France has frequently emphasized 'completely safe sex' – the systematic protection of all practices with all partners[1] – there is evidence to suggest that condom use and, in general, 'safer sex' are adopted to varying degrees. Our work also points to the diversity of AIDS prevention strategies used by gay men that go beyond simple condom use. These different options, whose underlying logic and efficacy need to be better understood, appear to be correlated with the social position of gay men in society as a whole as well as within the gay world itself.

For several reasons, our evaluation of these adaptations seeks to distance itself from public health debates that are pervaded by the notion of relapse (Ekstrand *et al.*, 1989). This concept, lacking in nuance to begin with, validates behaviours that are believed to constitute effective risk reduction practices and, conversely, condemns behaviour statistically linked to a return to risk practices. It appears, however, that any rigid distinction between 'safe' and 'unsafe' is over-simplified, whether it concerns groups of individuals confronted by the risk of AIDS, or time periods in the sexual career of an individual. This chapter analyses the ways in which gay and bisexual men who claim to have adapted their lifestyle to the risk of AIDS (and who are generally considered as practising HIV prevention), nevertheless report risking infection at least once during the year by not using a condom with a partner of unknown or different HIV status. Given the implications of this phenomenon for AIDS prevention, it is important for the social sciences to take it into account and, moreover, to try to explain it.

Until now, research on the factors influencing preventive behaviour has limited itself to studies of the adoption of condom use and the rules of 'safer sex'. The absence of a link between information about AIDS and preventive behaviour was an early finding in this field (Pollak *et al.*,1989). Furthermore, Michael Pollak pointed out in the early years of our studies that certain factors were highly correlated with the adoption of 'safer sex' by gay men; namely, personal proximity to the epidemic, elevated social and professional status coupled with a social acceptance of being homosexual, and a high degree of integration within the gay community (Pollak and Schiltz, 1987; Pollak, 1992). Recent French research on the general population also suggests that a prior awareness of risk is necessary for condom use (Spira *et al.*, 1993).

The major difficulty encountered in studying this question arises from the fact that even though much research tries to identify causal factors leading either to the adoption of preventive behaviour or to risk taking, social and psychological factors influence behaviour with respect to health and illness in a way that is frequently complex and unclear (Adam and Herzlich, 1994). A unified understanding of this problem thus remains to be developed, though attempts have been made to do this: Calvez, for example, has applied a culturalist approach to the problem of coping with risk (Douglas and Calvez, 1990). Likewise, the idea of there having been a 'rationalization' of sexuality underpins the work of Pollak from the end of the 1970s (Béjin and Pollak, 1977), an idea that the threat of AIDS has considerably redefined.

Not only are the factors leading to the adoption of preventive behaviour complex, but also the social sciences are relatively ill-equipped to explain risk taking by individuals who simultaneously claim to have adopted an effective strategy against the epidemic. This chapter is an initial attempt to explore these issues. In order to do so, we first sought to find out how gay men described the risks they took. The central question is thus: when an individual adopts a strategy of risk management, what happens to his awareness of risk? Depending on the strategy taken, a significant gap may exist between an individual's perception of risk and the actual risk as described by epidemiological criteria. Starting from our observation that risk assessment is highly subjective, we examine the effect that the belief in certain strategies can have on the individuals who follow them.

Specifically, we have chosen those individuals who have practiced unprotected anal intercourse with their non-regular sexual partners. We then examine their risk-management strategies to determine if they have under or over-declared their risk taking. Indeed, putting a risk management strategy into practice is not merely a method of reducing exposure to infection, it also strongly influences the way that a person perceives his exposure to AIDS. This influence, which we will analyse in detail, can be much stronger when a discourse validating certain feelings or certain forms of behaviour, including

2

'safer sex', accentuates its effects. In an effort to control AIDS, it is imperative to control the potential effects of any kind of overly categorical social discourse. Before developing these different points, we will briefly describe the study and the methodology adopted.

Procedure and Methodology

This study constitutes one of the elements of the research programme established by Michael Pollak. It analyses findings from a questionnaire survey conducted every year since 1985 in the gay press. The questionnaire is concerned primarily with sexuality, and oriented to the specific issue of AIDS. In addition to questions on socio-demographic characteristics (age, marital status, place of residence, profession, level of education), other questions establish the nature of respondents' social relations and whether they are more homosexual or more heterosexual. The principal objective of the survey is to identify the changes that the AIDS has brought about in the sexual life and social lives of those surveyed. The survey also identifies the behaviour and attitudes of the respondents *vis-à-vis* their health, with particular attention to HIV status. Finally, several questions access opinions about the status of gay and bisexual men and the social repercussions of the epidemic.

Using the gay press to collect data is not a neutral technique to adopt. In addition, having to return the questionnaire by post tends to bias the sample towards the most motivated respondents. Nevertheless, this mechanism (which constitutes a methodological and financial compromise), has permitted us to recruit rapidly and repeatedly a large number of respondents. The following analysis has been carried out using the 1991 and 1993 surveys in which 2000 and 3300 gay men, respectively, participated.

Although such a study cannot claim to be representative, the likely biases can be identified. First, we can compare the socio-demographic characteristics of those surveyed with statistics about single men in the same age group collected from the national census (Pollak *et al.*, 1986). This comparison indicates that our samples under-represent working-class individuals with limited education and over-represent university-educated professionals. As far as geographical distribution is concerned, our samples accurately represent the reference population with a slight over-representation of the Paris metropolitan area and also of areas containing fewer than 20,000 inhabitants. Thus, our study attracts not only those who are likely to be the most open about their homosexuality, but also those individuals living in smaller towns and in villages, who are more or less isolated from the rest of the gay world.

Government statistical indicators are not, however, the only ones that structure the gay population. Respondents' age at first sexual experience is also an indicator of potential bias in the sample. For the generation of men aged 25–45 years, our statistics coincide exactly with findings from the *Analyse des Comportements Sexuels en France* (ACSF) (Bozon, 1993); a nationwide study with a representative sample of 20,055 men and women. On the other hand, the youngest and the oldest members of our sample are sexually more precocious than their counterparts in the general population. Our method of recruiting is probably the cause of this difference. By using the gay press, we tend to select respondents whose sexuality plays an important role in their lives. This over-selection of the most sexually active men is that much greater as it concerns men at the beginning and end of their sexual career; precisely those age groups where the proportion of sexually inactive men is the highest.

Other indicators can also be taken into account. Relatively limited participation in gay and AIDS organizations shows that our sample is not limited to a core group of activists. Finally, in comparison with other studies using quota and snowball sampling techniques (Pollak and Schiltz, 1991), our respondents report a lower degree of acceptance of homosexuality, both by themselves and by others. The anonymity of the questionnaire and the absence of a face-to-face interview enable us to collect information from people who might ordinarily refuse to discuss their sexual preferences. Overall, it appears, as in other European studies (Bochow *et al.*, 1994), that a study using the gay press allows the description of the behaviour not only of the most socially and sexually active men, but also of bisexual and homosexual men who are reputedly more difficult to reach. Even though these latter groups constitute a minority within our sample, our study enables us to form hypotheses about them and to compare them to other groups of gay men. Hence, our goal is not to try to establish precise statistics concerning sexual behaviour. On the contrary, thanks to the large number of respondents, we can distinguish different groups of gay and bisexual men, each with different sexual practices and social characteristics. Our analysis is thus concerned with comparison between these groups. This kind of comparison also permits us to avoid the unanswerable question of whether those surveyed are in fact truthfully reporting their sexual practices.

Another distinctive feature of the study is the fact that the survey is conducted annually, thereby enabling the study of changes in behaviour. In order to make comparisons between different years, we have to be certain of the socio-demographic stability of our samples. Between 1985 and 1992, the magazine *Gai Pied* published the questionnaire and, as a result, the population remained extremely stable.[2] The disappearance of *Gai Pied* in 1993 forced us to modify the means of distribution. Since then, we have included the questionnaires in six gay magazines (*All Man, La Lettre de Gai Pied, Illico, Honcho, Lettres Gay, Rebel*). The choice of these periodicals originally reflected a desire to renew and enlarge the group participating in the survey. In 1993, this renewal was accomplished: 58.3 per cent of those responding did so for the first time (as opposed to 45.5 per cent in 1991). Although one would have expected considerable discontinuity in the 1993 sample, the socio-demographics of those surveyed in 1993 are entirely comparable with the characteristics of the preceding surveys, except that the 1993 population is younger, as was hoped (the average age of the sample declined from 34.9 years in 1991 to 33.4 years in 1993). This stability is probably due to the fact that *Gai Pied* itself had a diverse but progressively ageing readership. Thanks to the stability of the socio-demographic structure, this annual cycle of observations provides an overview of changes in sexual behaviour since our first study 10 years ago (Pollak and Schiltz, 1991; Schiltz, 1993).

Strategies of Adaptation

In order to evaluate gay men's reactions to the AIDS epidemic, we began by asking if they had ever taken precautions to prevent infection since its beginning. In 1985, only 44 per cent of those surveyed declared that they had taken preventive measures to avoid HIV infection; by 1988, however, this rate had levelled off at over 80 per cent. To this group of men who have modified their behaviour – the vast majority of the respondents – we must add in 1993 the 11.1 per cent who declare that they have always practised a form of 'safer sex'. This group generally consists of young men who began their sexual life after condom use had become more or less the norm. In 1993, the increase in the percentage of those who are 'already safe' is also due, at least in part, to a sample which is simply younger. Thus, with the exception of a small minority (3.8 per cent) who declare that they have not modified their sexual behavior in spite of the risk taken – whether it be by choice or because of the difficulties inherent in such a change – the risk of AIDS is now widely taken into account by gay men. The question is then: how exactly have gay men modified their behaviour?[3]

Condom Use

Condom use reflects a major adaptation to the risk of AIDS among gay men. Since 1989, condom use has stabilized at a high level, with three-quarters of those surveyed describing themselves as users (see Table 1.1). Statistics concerning overall condom use mask variations in use that depend both on the type of sexual practices and on the nature of the sexual partner. With casual or non-regular partners, prudence is the rule. Not only do dangerous sexual practices tend to be generally excluded, but when practised they are more protected. This is as true for fellatio as it is for anal penetration.

Although only a minority of those surveyed use condoms for fellatio,[5] the percentages increase slightly for non-regular partners: more than a third of

Table 1.1 Condom use[4]

Year	1985	1986	1987	1988	1989	1990	1991	1992	1993
Sample size	992	1189	1225	1500	1497	1997	1994	893	3275
Total use (%)	5.6	35.1	58.4	61.4	76.5	74.4	74.0	73.6	76.9

those surveyed use a condom 'sometimes' or 'always' for oral-genital contact. Likewise, fellatio without ejaculation is becoming more common. With casual partners, 83.9 per cent of those surveyed in 1991 and 87.7 per cent in 1993 systematically avoid receiving semen in the mouth.

We note not only that 25.8 per cent in 1991 and 18.7 per cent in 1993 of the respondents avoided anal penetration altogether, but those continuing to practice it protect themselves more (see Table 1.2). Thus in 1993, 81.5 per cent of those responding have either abandoned penetration (18.7 per cent) or use condoms during every act with a casual partner (63.8 per cent). The

Table 1.2 Nature and protection of sexual practices

Year	Regular partner		Non-regular partner(s)	
	1991 (%)	1993 (%)	1991 (%)	1993 (%)
Fellatio				
number	1366	1793	1504	2398
no fellatio	1.8	1.7	6.3	3.4
always protected	6.6	5.4	13.2	12.8
sometimes protected	10.5	7.4	22.9	26.5
never protected	81.1	85.6	57.6	57.3
	$\chi^2=12.5$	p<0.01	$\chi^2=22.1$	p<0.01
Ejaculation in the mouth				
number	1427	1897	1546	2489
no fellatio	1.7	1.6	6.1	3.3
never	72.8	72.4	83.9	87.7
sometimes	21.2	21.9	8.5	8.1
always	4.3	4.1	1.5	1.0
	$\chi^2=$ns	p>0.05	$\chi^2=21.6$	p<0.01
Anal penetration				
number	1418	1869	1517	2463
no penetration	12.5	10.6	25.8	18.7
always protected	37.2	37.0	52.9	63.8
sometimes protected	12.7	9.9	11.5	9.6
never protected	37.7	42.5	9.8	7.9
	$\chi^2=128$	p<0.01	$\chi^2=478$	p<0.01

global figure falls to 47.6 per cent in relationships with a regular partner. Between 1991 and 1993 we note that the difference in protection with non-regular and with regular partners becomes more pronounced. The preceding description shows that there exists a diversity of condom use. It is important not only to understand the logic behind these variations, but also to recognize that condom use is not the only risk management strategy adopted.

In order to examine these other strategies, we asked respondents to characterize the behaviour they had adopted for coping with the risk of AIDS by choosing from among a number of possibilities.[6] Although a small number of men indicated no chosen method of prevention,[7] the responses of the rest of the respondents enable us to identify the different risk-management strategies adopted by gay men. In addition to what we call the category of 'maintaining risky behaviour' (strategy 0), which groups together those who declare themselves unable or unwilling to modify their sexual practices despite the risks, three major types of strategies appear in the pattern of responses.

First, some individuals believe that they can reduce their exposure to infection by applying what we call the 'selection and avoidance' strategy (strategy 1). These individuals reduce their number of partners, choose their partners by appearance, avoid allegedly dangerous pick-up spots, and even seek regular relationships. Second, over the years, a strategy based on 'shared responsibility' (strategy 2) has developed. Under this rubric we place both those men who have a monogamous relationship (strategy 2a) and those who have decided to have unprotected sex with their stable partner following an agreement systematically to protect themselves during 'extra-conjugal' relations (strategy 2b, henceforth referred to as the 'shared responsibility within an open couple' strategy). Finally, the 'protectionist strategy' (strategy 3) groups together those gay men who have opted for 'safer sex'; in other words, either systematically protected sex or the abandonment of the most dangerous practices.

Presented in this way, the different strategies appear independent. This is not, however, always the case: different individuals often report a pattern of behaviour that combines elements belonging to different options. Confronted with this situation, we have created a hierarchy among the different practices, ordered by inclusion: strategy 3 can include strategy 2, which can include strategy 1. This hierarchy reflects the level of protection afforded by each strategy according to 'objective' criteria relating to the risk of infection. When an individual reports using several strategies, it is always the most effective strategy that takes precedence, unless he admits to maintaining risky behaviour. In that case, continuing to live at risk excludes any other declaration. Thus, the adoption of protective measures takes precedence over prevention based on shared responsibility. The reduction of situations of exposure ('selection and avoidance') is cited as the adopted strategy only in the absence of any other. Hence, a respondent with a monogamous relationship who

Table 1.3 Coping or avoidance strategies

Year	1991 (%)	1993 (%)
Number	1994	3275
no strategy	5.2	1.6
maintenance of risky behaviour (0)	5.7	3.8
selectionist strategy (1)	8.3	8.1
shared responsibility strategy: fidelity (2a)	5.7	7.3
shared responsibility strategy: open couple (2b)	3.9	6.2
protectionist strategy (3)	71.2	72.9
	χ^2=84.9;	p>0.01

systematically practices 'safer sex' will be classified as having a 'protectionist' strategy. On the other hand, someone who takes only protective measures for sexual relations outside of his regular relationship and who has, moreover, reduced the number of partners is classified as having a strategy of shared responsibility. This classification enables us to determine the relative importance of the different strategies adopted by gay men confronting the risks of AIDS.

It is apparent from Table 1.3 that the vast majority of gay men (72.9 per cent in 1993) have opted for a 'protectionist' strategy. As we have seen, abandoning penetration is an option chosen only by a minority of men within this group. It is thus the systematic use of condoms that best describes the preventive measures taken. 'Shared responsibility' has been adopted by 13.6 per cent of the gay men surveyed.[8] Finally, despite the prevention campaigns, a minority of men (8.1 per cent) have opted for a strategy based on 'selection and avoidance'.[9] Table 1.3 also illustrates significant changes in strategies between 1991 and 1993. While the number of men who follow a strategy of 'selection and avoidance' remains stable, there is a reduction in the number of men who state that they have 'no strategy' or who 'maintain risks'. Over the same period, there is a large increase among those subscribing to the strategy of 'shared responsibility within a couple'.[10] It is possible to describe those reporting different strategies as 'clusters', each of which has particular social characteristics linked either to their position in society as a whole, or within the gay world. The cluster of men who maintain risky behaviour is composed mainly of bisexual men who have had multiple female partners during the year, and gay men of relatively limited education and socio-economic standing. In their responses to our survey, they talk of their powerlessness to change their sexual habits, whether it be with non-regular or with regular partners.

The cluster of men who follow a 'selectionist' strategy and seek to avoid those sexual encounters considered to be at highest risk, is mainly composed of gay men who live comparatively marginalized lives with respect to the rest of the gay community. To the extent that when they go to gay pick-up spots, they do so secretly. Their socio-economic standing and level of education also tend to be lower than other groups. As a result of being seen as too old or too young, they may be experiencing a period of difficulty in their sexual career. They also tend to participate more than others in a heterosexual lifestyle. This set of factors thus adds up to a marginalization of these men from the gay world. In addition, we observe both that these men have sex infrequently and that the epidemic does not touch their day to day lives. To sum up, with respect to the gay world in which they participate, but also due to their unfavourable status in society as a whole, they suffer from multiple marginalization. This is due to social (low socio-economic standing, limited education), geographic (distance from a gay social centre), as well as sexual (they are too old or too young, bisexual, or involved in a heterosexual lifestyle), and emotional (tenuous social relationships, the influence of a heterosexual social milieu – female partners or dependence on a family – that disapproves of homosexuality) factors.

A third cluster of men are those whom we call the 'pure protectionists'. Generally 35–45 years old, these men systematically protect themselves at every sexual encounter, without, however, otherwise modifying their sexual practices or their lifestyles, which are often characterized by a large number of partners. They themselves have personally felt the effects of the epidemic (friends and lovers who are HIV positive, sick, or dead) and those forming part of a couple are, more often than for other groups of gay men, HIV positive with a history of sexually transmitted infection. For those who live alone, the epidemic is primarily experienced through their sexual partners.

The strategy of 'shared responsibility' is adopted by two relatively distinct groups of men. One group is composed of those who have resorted to fidelity as a means of maintaining a sex life without the constraint of 'safer sex' (these individuals report regular unprotected anal intercourse). This group is clearly distinguished from another set of gay men who live as couples, but are not monogamous and protect themselves only in their non-regular encounters. The latter group is composed mostly of upper-middle-class gay men. Among gay men in general, it is this latter group who puts into practise the most complex strategies of risk management. They adapt to the risk of AIDS by modifying both their lifestyle and their sexual behaviour. They have a limited number of partners, and with their non-regular partners they have modified their sexual practices. More often than for any other group they have abandoned penetration; for fellatio they use condoms and avoid ejaculation in the mouth.

Risk Evaluation

Having described these risk-management strategies, we can go on to obtain a broad overview of the risks associated with each of them in terms of becoming infected or infecting someone else. Overall, a significant number of gay men continue to expose themselves to risk. When we combine the minority of men who have chosen a 'selection and avoidance' strategy,[11] those who maintain risky behaviour,[12] and finally, those with 'no declared strategy', we estimate that 19 per cent in 1991 and 14 per cent in 1993 are situated in a 'risk zone'. For the remaining gay men, those who state having a 'protectionist' or 'shared responsibility' strategy, we must examine more closely the coherence of their chosen strategy and, as we shall see, a number of indicators attest to their continued exposure to risk.[14]

Any evaluation of such risk must take into account anal penetration.[15] Unlike heterosexual sex, where vaginal penetration is almost universally practised (Spira *et al.*, 1993), not all homosexual contact includes anal intercourse. Nevertheless, the men in our survey remain very attached to this form of sexual activity: only about 10 per cent of them have abandoned penetration with their regular partners and only about one quarter with their non-regular partners. Hence, we believe that the most reliable index of risk is based on an evaluation of the practice of unprotected anal penetration with a partner of different or unknown HIV status, henceforth called unsafe sex (*pénétration à risque*). Clearly, discordant HIV status is not only possible in such circumstances,[16] but may have profound implications for the participants.

Having chosen to limit ourselves to the study of non-regular encounters, we have proceeded in two different ways to evaluate the exposure to risk. The first is based on 'objective' indicators provided by responents' detailed descriptions of their sexual practices with non-regular partners. The second is more 'subjective' since it is based on each respondent's own evaluation of the risks incurred. Each time that a respondent has reported practising penetration that was not systematically protected with a non-regular partner, we say that he has risked infection. Indeed, in the context of non-regular encounters, the participants are usually unable to take advantage of any reliable knowledge of their partner's HIV status. Based on this first criterion, it appears that 21.3 per cent in 1991 and 17.5 per cent in 1993 who engage in casual sex continue to take major risks. This indicator is illustrated in Table 1.2: 'penetration protected occasionally or never with casual partners'.

We have, in addition, asked those surveyed if they have engaged in unprotected anal penetration at least once with a casual partner whose HIV status was unknown. The question was thus approached directly and the answer left to the judgement of those surveyed. Their responses provide a second indicator of risk: 16.6 per cent of the 1991 respondents and 14.6

per cent of the 1993 respondents claim to have had anal intercourse with a non-regular partner of unknown or different HIV status, regardless of their practices with their stable partner.[17] If we compare these two indicators of risk, they do not match exactly. The rate of reported unsafe sex (*pénétration à risque*) declared for the latter index (16.6 per cent in 1991 and 14.6 per cent in 1993) is markedly lower than what the first index would lead us to believe. (Indeed, 21.3 per cent of sexually active respondents in 1991, and 17.5 per cent of sexually active respondents in 1993 indicate that they have engaged in anal intercourse 'occasionally' or 'never' protected with non-regular partners.)

That this latter index is lower would imply that in responding to the question 'In the last 12 months, have you engaged in unprotected anal penetration at least once with a (casual) partner whose HIV status you did not know or whose HIV status was different from your own?', the respondents failed to report accurately their history of unprotected anal intercourse. Therefore, not all unprotected anal penetration with casual partners is considered risky by those surveyed. In this context, the formulation of this question has evidently given rise to inconsistent answers. It turns out that the differences between the estimation of risk based on unsystematic protection on the one hand, and the declarations of risk by gay and bisexual men on the other vary even more when we consider specific groups of gay men. Thus, in other words, the men surveyed do not all demonstrate the same degree of risk awareness. As we sought to best understand the factors that could induce these differences in the perception of risk, it appeared to us that the declared strategies played a determining role.

Risk Awareness and Reported Strategies

In order to determine if those surveyed have a tendency to over-declare or to under-declare the risk of infection they have incurred, we used two different procedures. First, we examined a population of individuals who exposed themselves to a comparable risk, in order to determine if these men had an identical awareness of risk or if there existed a disparity in their attitudes. Second, we compared sub-groups of individuals who had been exposed to differential risk and determined the way in which these men perceived that difference. Our starting hypothesis was that the level of awareness of risk of gay men varies as a function of the strategies of adaptation to the epidemic to which they subscribe.

Comparable level of exposure to risk and corresponding variability in the awareness of risk

We first compare the level of risk declaration by individuals who have opted for different strategies, but whom the analysis has shown to have comparable exposure to risk. In order to do this, we have eliminated those men who have considerably reduced their objective exposure to risk; namely, those who are sexually inactive, those who do not practise penetration, those who always use a condom, and those who have been in a monogamous relationship and have had only one partner all year.[18] Those men retained in the analysis (n=573 out of a total of 2670) are those who are sexually active outside of a primary relationship; in other words, 21.5 per cent of the total. All of them 'irregularly' or 'never' use condoms during anal intercourse with non-regular partners thus exposing themselves to that risk of infection. Although certain among them may claim to have a 'shared responsibility' (Strategy 2b most often) or 'protectionist' strategy, it is not strictly applied. Significant differences appear between those who declare a strategy of risk management and those who do not.

We know that risk increases with the number of partners, (Schiltz, 1993). We note, however, that the variations in Table 1.4 are not simply the result of the number of partners for the different groups. Indeed, although the 'selectionists' generally have fewer partners than the practitioners of 'safer sex', it is the 'selectionists' who report a greater risk exposure. Furthermore, it appears that within each strategy, the rates of declaration of risk grow as a function of the number of partners, but the global differences between them remain the same. Indeed, for the same number of partners, it is always those following a couple-based strategy who report the lowest risk and those following a 'selectionist' strategy who report the highest. The 'protectionist' strategy occupies a place between these two extremes.

In order to interpret Table 1.4, we use the incidence of unsafe sex

Table 1.4 *Rate of declaration of at least one act of unprotected anal penetration with a non-regular partner of unknown or different HIV status by men who practice penetration that is 'irregularly' or 'never' protected with casual partners, according to the strategy they claim to follow*

Strategy	no declared risk (%)	declared risk (%)	
number	n=179	n=220	number
maintenance of risk	30.2	69.8	n=53
selectionist strategy	33.3	66.7	n=75
shared responsibility	70.2	29.8	n=47
protectionist strategy	47.5	52.5	n=221
	$\chi^2=23.9$	p<0.01	

(*pénétration à risque*) for those maintaining risk behaviour (i.e. 69.8 per cent) as a baseline. From this reference point, we observe that the 'protectionists' and those who have adopted the 'shared responsibility' strategy under-estimate the risk incurred (their rates being 52.5 per cent and 29.8 per cent respectively). Our sample size is too small to pursue a more in-depth statistical analysis. It appears, nevertheless, that the strategy based on 'conjugal' fidelity leads to a more pronounced under-estimation of risk than the strategy of protection for extra-conjugal relations.

The preceding remarks show that for some gay men, subscribing to a 'protectionist' or 'shared responsibility' strategy, albeit not strictly applied, is a 'myth of reality maintenance' (Berger and Luckmann, 1967) in as much as it leads to an under-estimation of risk. The normative validation of 'safer sex' among gay men undoubtedly contributes to imposing a model of safer relationships. This validation, like the belief in 'conjugal' fidelity, can nevertheless have a detrimental effect by inordinately reassuring those who evidently do expose themselves to the risk of infection.

In 1993, 'selectionists' reporting of risk is statistically indistinguishable from those who acknowledge maintaining risks (66.7 per cent versus 69.8 per cent). Research has repeatedly indicated that some gay men were employing strategies which they believed effective, but were completely ineffective from an epidemiological point of view. Several findings lead us to believe that the 'selection and avoidance' strategy has lost credibility over the last few years. We know that there exist both 'pure selectionists' as well as individuals who employ either the 'shared responsibility' or 'protectionist' strategies while at the same time 'selecting' their partners and avoiding certain pick up spots.[19] When we do an overall analysis of these different groups – the results of which appear in Table 1.5 – we note that between 1991 and 1993, the proportion of men who follow the 'selection and avoidance' strategy, be it exclusively or in combination with other strategies, diminishes significantly.[20]

Table 1.5 illustrates, however, that the drop in the number of men who employ the 'selection and avoidance' strategy is significantly greater among those who also follow a more effective strategy.[21] We can thus conclude that the 'selection and avoidance' strategy has lost credibility for those men who know how to manage risk. Pure selectionists base their method of HIV prevention on the avoidance of allegedly risky situations, and in particular, HIV positive partners. Nevertheless, they are more readily disposed to seek information from partners that will allow them to identify someone who is HIV positive (24.4 per cent versus 16.1 per cent for the survey population as a whole). This may be evidence of a certain uneasiness on the part of those men who, though seeking to cope with the epidemic by avoiding HIV-positive partners, do not have confidence in their own criteria for recognition. The 'pure selectionists', who are generally characterized (by limited social resour-ces and marginality from the rest of the gay world, are far from unconcerned

Table 1.5 Evolution of the possible choices of selection and avoidance in the different risk management strategies

Year number	1991 n=1994			1993 n=3275		
	select (%)	share responsi-bility (%)	protect (%)	select (%)	share responsi-bility (%)	protect (%)
reduce the number of partners	54.8	55.7	46.5	41.7	21.4	21.0
choice of partners	49.4	28.4	40.0	42.9	12.6	18.0
abandon certain pick-up spots	31.5	34.9	24.5	22.9	12.4	13.5
seek a stable relationship	48.2	42.2	47.4	62.8	20.5	27.1

by the risks their lifestyle incurs (Table 1.4). They may maintain this strategy because of an incapacity to otherwise cope with risk. As we will see, we encounter a similar phenomenon when we study the case of men who only rarely use a condom despite continued exposure to risk.

Variability of awareness of risk according to the more or less systematic protection of anal intercourse

We have shown that individuals in situations of comparable risk interpret their situations in different ways. It may likewise be the case that interpretation of situations of increasing risk does not systematically correspond to risk defined from an epidemiological standpoint. In other words, it may be that greater exposure to infection does not necessarily translate into a greater sense of risk. In order to explore this phenomenon, we have chosen to focus on the use of condoms by men practising anal penetration with non-regular partners. If the reports of risk objectively describe the exposure to risk, those practising penetration that is 'always protected' should declare less risk than those for whom penetration is only 'occasionally protected', which group should, likewise, declare less risk than those practising penetration that is 'never protected.'

Table 1.6 shows, however, that reports of unsafe sex (*pénétration à risque*) is at its maximum for gay men who practise 'rarely protected' penetration and not for those who never protect themselves. It appears that instead of enjoying a sense of increased security, the group of occasional condom users has a more acute sense of risk.

The ACSF study of the general population has also shown that occasional condom users experience a greater awareness of danger than others (Spira *et al.*, 1993). The authors explain this by the fact that condom use is the result of a prior sense of increased risk. We think that the occasional use of a

Table 1.6 Percentage of those surveyed who declare unprotected penetration at least once with casual partner(s) unknown or different HIV status, according to the degree of protection

Year	1991	1993
	(%)	(%)
number	1602	2385
no penetration	5.4	2.7
penetration, always protected	15.9	13.5
penetration, rarely protected	64.0	69.3
penetration, never protected	43.9	32.3

condom may likewise have an effect on the individual's awareness of risk. When such use is irregular, it introduces a notion of risk in the sexual life of the person concerned: not only must he make a decision about whether to protect himself each time he has sex, but the condom itself may act as a physical reminder of the risk of AIDS.

In order to better understand this phenomenon, one may characterize the group of sometime condom users by their strategic behaviour. The majority of these men maintain risks or claim to be 'selectionists'. Even though they are condom users, these men have not made condom use a point of reference for their sexual practices. Their cognitive universe has not been reorganized around a belief in the effectiveness of this method of risk management. As a result, the individuals experience a 'loss of bearings' and henceforth an increased perception of risk.

Conclusions

At the end of this analysis, it is clear that gay men have massively adopted 'safer sex'. We observe, however, that some men, frequently those who are socially disadvantaged in some way, maintain risky behaviour or employ ineffective strategies. Far from being 'unconcerned', these men experience difficulties due to their lack of social resources and to their limited 'homosexual competence'. The task of prevention cannot be limited to encouraging condom use alone. As AIDS is a problem that has no short term solution, we should concern ourselves henceforth with improving the quality of life of these men. Support from society as a whole, an acceptance of self, and a sense of well-being may appear to be too abstract as the basis for a policy of AIDS prevention; all the same, they do lead to better risk management.

In order to make prevention more effective, it is also necessary to move beyond the promotion of a single model of 'safer sex'. The adaptations induced by the risk of AIDS are more complex than might be presupposed by a 'safer sex' dogma that advocates systematic protection for all practices and for all partners. By no means are all of these adaptations ineffective. If the large majority of gay men have opted for the 'protectionist' strategy (72.9 per cent in 1993), a strategy of 'shared responsibility' in the context of a regular relationship has nevertheless been adopted by 13.6 per cent of those surveyed. Of this latter group of men, 7.3 per cent declare themselves to be monogamous and the rest (6.3 per cent) have chosen a strategy of 'shared responsibility in an open couple'. Between 1991 and 1993, we note an increase in the couple-based strategies that rely on the use of the HIV test. Rather than ignoring the existence of this diversity of approaches, prevention campaigns should take them into account. The point is to help gay men to adopt and improve the method of risk management that best corresponds to their lifestyle. This is all the more urgent as the objective of zero risk appears today to be unattainable.

Indeed, given the non-negligible rate of unsafe sex (*pénétration à risque*), that characterizes the 'sexual market', zero risk remains a Utopian goal. This difficulty does not uniquely concern those individuals whose behaviour remains unchanged in spite of the epidemic. It likewise applies, albeit to a lesser degree, to those who claim to subscribe to effective strategies. The idea of relapse is inadequate to explain this phenomenon: we know that events labelled as 'risky' and 'risk free' do not necessarily correspond to successive periods in time, but may exist simultaneously in a larger time frame. One of the central questions that has informed our analysis is to know how gay men themselves account for this phenomenon. We can clearly distinguish two poles of opinion.

Those individuals who adopt strategies that are epidemiologically ineffective, such as 'selection and avoidance', are not fooled by their own behaviour. On the contrary, they have a stronger awareness of risk than other gay men. The second pole, on the other hand, is composed of individuals who follow reputedly effective strategies (whether they be 'protectionist' or 'shared responsibility'), but who have engaged in unsafe sex (*pénétration à risque*) as a result of a lax application of their chosen strategy. We observe, in their case, that these men have a tendency to under-report their risk of infection. One may think that this minimization of risk constitutes a form of adaptation to the epidemic: gay men are not limiting themselves merely to applying technical rules to avoid infection, they are attempting to maintain their participation in the 'sexual market', and at the same time attempt to reduce their sense of danger. This minimization results from a belief in the effectiveness of a strategy that they have adopted and relies on some type of 'myth of reality maintenance' (Berger and Luckmann, 1967). The fact that some gay men have confidence in the couple as a means of protection has certainly led to the credibility of the 'shared responsibility' strategies. We have shown, however, that certain 'myths of reality maintenance' seem to come into play and at the same time distort the guidelines of 'safer sex'. The fact that some gay men consider themselves to be safe – although this is not always the case – allows them to under-estimate the risks they actually take. Hence, the normative validation of 'safer sex' can, for some groups of gay men, produce entirely unexpected effects.

The reality perceived by individuals is thus not objective fact; on the contrary, as Berger and Luckman had stressed (1967), it is a social construction founded upon the ideology and the beliefs shared by the members of a certain social group.[22] Prevention campaigns should take this phenomenon into account and incorporate into their methods of communication the manner in which different subpopulations of gay and bisexual men perceive the risk of AIDS. Those men who are the most worried about AIDS must be reassured and reconciled with their own sexuality in the context of the safer-sex model. Moreover, it is necessary to encourage those men unduly confident in safer-sex or in a couple-based strategy to be more prudent in their actions.

Acknowledgements

Text translated from the French by Francis Kelly. The authors would like to thank Nathalie Bajos, Michael Bochow and Peter Davies for their assistance during the preparation of this Chapter.

Notes

1 This method of risk management has been advocated by the AIDS prevention community as the means of dealing with the epidemic that is best suited to gay men.

2 Founded in 1979, this publication had a dominant position in the gay press up until its closure in 1992.

3 Just over two per cent of respondents had no sexual partners during the year. We categorize these men as 'sexually inactive' and excluded them from the analysis.

4 The percentage in parenthesis indicates the result of an open question from the 1985 questionnaire. It is thus difficult to compare this result with the other statistics in the table.

5 As far as fellatio is concerned, those responsible for prevention in France encourage condom use in general and recommend against ejaculation in the mouth without a condom.

6 Multiple choice responses came from the following list: (1) I have reduced the number of my sexual partners (2) I choose my partners cautiously, based on their appearance; (3) I have given up certain pick-up spots; (4) I practise safe-sex; (5) I limit myself to mutual masturbation and caresses; (6) I'm looking for a stable relationship; (7) My partner and I have a monogamous relationship; (8) I practise safe-sex outside of my stable relationship.

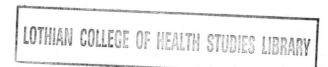

7   5.2 per cent in 1991 and 1.6 per cent in 1993.

8   'Conjugal fidelity' has been adopted as a risk management strategy by 7.3 per cent of those surveyed, or 240 people; 'shared responsibility in an open couple' has been adopted by 6.3 per cent of the respondents or 204 people.

9   By way of comparison, in the heterosexual French population 'partner selection' is the predominant way of coping with the risk of AIDS (Spira *et al.*, 1993). In this population, however, the number of HIV positive individuals is comparatively low. In 1993, 17% of our respondents were HIV positive. Taking an HIV test is very common in France: 81.4% of respondents had taken the HIV test at least once (Schiltz and Adam, 1995).

10 This increase is not due to the fact that the population is younger. For those under 25 years of age, the percentage following a 'shared responsibility' strategy increases from 9.6% to 14% from 1991 to 1993. For those over 25, this percentage increases from 9.3% to 13,5%. Thus, over this period, the statistical difference remains constant for those over and under 25.

11 8.3 per cent in 1991 and 8.1 per cent in 1993.

12 5.7 per cent in 1991 and 3.8 per cent in 1993.

13 5.2 per cent in 1991 and 1.6 per cent in 1993.

14 Among men who declare themselves monogamous, we find 5 per cent of those who practise penetration with non-regular partners that is 'occasionally' or 'never' protected. This percentage is 10 per cent for those who follow a 'protectionist' strategy, and 18 per cent for those who follow a strategy of protection for 'extra-conjugal' encounters.

15 In France, fellatio is also considered to be a practice that theoretically carries a risk of infection, though the risk may be very small. For study purposes, we prefer to consider only the principal risk practice, anal penetration.

16 Approximately 17 per cent of our respondents are HIV positive.

17 Our observations indicate, furthermore, that 10.2 per cent of the respondents in 1992 and 9.2 per cent in 1993 have had 'unprotected anal intercourse' at least once with a regular partner of unknown or different HIV-status, whether or not it be only with this person. This problem, which merits further attention, will not be discussed further here.

18 Given that we are interested in non-regular encounters, those individuals we classify as sexually inactive and those in a couple declaring only one partner in the year are henceforth excluded from the analysis.

19 The different elements making up the 'selection and avoidance' strategy are: reduction of the number of partners, avoiding certain pick-up spots, choosing partners on the basis of appearance, or looking for a stable relationship as a way to avoid AIDS.

20 For our entire sample.

21 In 1991, 31.5 per cent of the 'selectionists' had abandoned certain gay pick-up spots; in 1993, this figure fell to 22.9 per cent. The same drop can be found among the respondents employing a 'shared responsibility' strategy (34.9 per cent versus 12.4 per cent) or a 'protectionist' strategy (24.5 per cent versus 13.5 per cent). These reductions can be found for all the elements of the 'selectionist' strategy.

22 These results, which indicate on effect of the adopted strategy on the level of awareness of risk, cannot however be applied identically to all gay men. Our data,

show that HIV-positive gay men have an awareness of risk considerably more acute than their HIV negative brethren. In a sense, they themselves 'embody' an awareness of risk in that they apply the criteria of public health to evaluate their own level of exposure to risk. One may hypothesize that being HIV positive is, in general, a sufficiently dramatic experience to destroy any unfounded belief in the effectiveness of a strategy of protection (Schiltz and Adam, 1995).

References

ADAM P. and HERZLICH, C. (1994) *Sociologie de la maladie et de la médecine*, Collection Sociologie 128, Paris: Nathan-Université.

BEJIN, A. and POLLAK, M. (1977) 'La rationalisation de la sexualité', *Cahiers Internationaux de Sociologie*, **62**.

BERGER, P.L. and LUCKMANN, T. (1967) *The Social Construction of Reality: a treatise of sociology of knowledge*, Garden City, NY: Doubleday.

BOCHOW, M., CHIAROTTI, F., DAVIES, P., DUBOIS-ARBER, F. DÜR, W., FOUCHARD, J., *et al.* (1994) Sexual behaviour of gay and bisexual men in eight European countries', *AIDS Care*, **6** (5), 533–49.

BOZON, M. (1993) 'L'entrée dans la sexualité adulte: le premier rapport et ses suites. Du calendrier aux attitudes', *Population*, **48**(5), 1317–52.

DOUGLAS, M. and CALVEZ M. (1990) 'The self as risk taker: a cultural theory of contagion in relation to AIDS', *Sociological Review*, **38**, 445–65.

EKSTRAND, M.L., STALL, R.D., COATES, T.J. and MCKUSICK, L. (1989) 'Risky Sex, Relapse, The Next Challenge for AIDS Prevention Programmes: the AIDS behavioural research project', Poster presented at the Fifth International Conference on AIDS, Montreal, TD08.

POLLAK, M., DAB, W. and MOATTI, J.-P. (1989) 'Systèmes de réaction au SIDA et action préventive', *Sciences Sociales et Santé*, **7**(1), 111–40.

POLLAK, M. (1992) 'Assessing AIDS prevention among male homo- and bisexuals', in PACCAUD, F., VADER, J.-P. and GUTZWILLER, F. (Eds) *Assessing AIDS Prevention*, Basel: Birkhauser Verlag.

POLLAK, M. and SCHILTZ M.-A. (1987) 'Identité sociale et gestion d'un risque de santé', *Actes de la Recherche en Sciences Sociales*, **68**, 77–102.

POLLAK, M. and SCHILTZ, M.A. (1991) *Six Années d'Enquêtes sur Les Homo- et Bisexuels Masculins Face au Sida*, Paris: Rapport à l'Agence Nationale de Recherche sur le Sida.

POLLAK, M., SCHILTZ, M.A. and LAURINDO, L. (1986) 'Les homosexuels face à l'épidémie du SIDA', *Revue Epidémiologique et Santé Publique*, **34**, 143–53.

SCHILTZ, M.A. (1993) *Les Homosexuels Masculins Face au sida: Enquêtes 1991–1992*. Paris: Rapport l'Agence Nationale de Recherche sur le Sida.

SCHILTZ, M.A. and ADAM, P. (1995) *Les homosexuels face an sida: enquête 1993 sur les modes de vie et la gestion du risque VIH*, Paris: Rapport à l'Agence Nationale de Recherche sur le sida et à la Direction Générale de la Santé.

SPIRA, A., BAJOS, N. and le groupe ACSF (1993) *Les Comportements Sexuels en France*, Paris: La Documentation Française.

Chapter 2

HIV-Related Discrimination in Medical Teaching Texts

Catherine Waldby, Susan Kippax and June Crawford

Investigations into the phenomenon of HIV-related discrimination often observe that it seems to reach its greatest intensity within medical institutions and in the practice of health care professionals. Gostin (1992) in his survey of HIV-related discrimination litigation in the US, maintains that other sites of discrimination, in education and the workplace for example, have witnessed a lessening of discriminatory practice as the epidemic progresses, and that 'complaints about discrimination in health care, nursing, and social services have predominated in recent years' (Gostin 1992: 159). The New South Wales Anti-Discrimination Board Report on AIDS-related discrimination similarly notes that discrimination is 'most consistently and extensively reported in [the area] of health care' both in Australia and internationally, and is documented in the services of 'general practitioners, hospitals, surgeons, dentists, and allied health professionals' (NSW Anti-Discrimination Board, 1992: 30).

In spite of this intensification of discriminatory practices at medical sites, medical knowledge itself tends to be posed as the antidote to, or opposite of, discriminatory ideas in the social science and policy literature that documents HIV-related discrimination. The Anti-Discrimination Board's report cited above provides a good example of this assumption, when it states,

> Surveys of the attitudes of health care professionals suggest a high level of anxiety about HIV and AIDS, and of discomfort about the people with whom the disease is most identified, and a preparedness to discriminate in ways which conflict ... with scientific knowledge about the disease.
>
> (NSW Anti-Discrimination Board, 1992: 30)

This exemption of medical knowledge from suspicion within the discriminatory model of power relationships seems rather unsatisfactory in the light of a growing literature which demonstrates that medical discourse is implicated in complex ways in the maintenance of HIV-related discriminatory practices. The work of Epstein (1988), Treichler (1988), Patton (1990), Bolton (1992) and Oppenheimer (1992), for example, all trace the process of the social construction of the disease 'AIDS' and the extent to which medical science relied upon unexamined, and often moralistic, ideas about homosexuality and other kinds of sexual and racial difference in order to make sense of the disease HIV/AIDS.

In order to consider further the relationship between discriminatory practice and medical knowledge, this chapter examines the representation of HIV/AIDS in medical teaching texts currently used in medical degree courses at two universities in Sydney, Australia. The nine textbooks examined here are used primarily in third and fourth year undergraduate medical courses, in the areas of immunology and the microbiology of infectious diseases, where HIV/AIDS is primarily located in the medical curriculum.

The representation of HIV/AIDS in medical textbooks can be considered to inform our study of two things. First, it simply indicates the nature of the knowledge of HIV/AIDS at the disposal of the present generation of internists and novice doctors. Beyond its immediate pedagogic circulation, however, textbook representations serve as a more general guide to the current consensus of understanding about HIV/AIDS within the bio-medical professions. As Fleck (1979) points out in his discussion of the relationship between journal science and textbook science, the textbook presents its material as proven factual knowledge, as the introduction to the novice of what is considered to be established and no longer open to significant question. For this reason textbooks can be read as indicative of professional consensus, the knowledge of HIV/AIDS which is not considered to be disputable. While we cannot verify that any individual doctor or paramedical professional will have such knowledge at their immediate disposal, nevertheless it forms the generally circulating body of knowledge and assumptions that health care workers can draw upon.

These textbooks have been investigated for two levels of discriminatory discourse. The first is an explicit level, the use of overtly discriminatory language and concepts in relation to people associated with HIV/AIDS in some way. The second is an implicit or systemic level of discourse, where certain aspects of the conceptualization of HIV/AIDS feed into discriminatory ideas.

It is important to note that in developing a critique of this medical discourse we do not wish to suggest that the bio-medical account is wrong or illusory. It is possible to consider this account as accurate in certain ways, but to nevertheless critically investigate its assumptions and the unacknowledged metaphoric systems through which it is thought. As Treichler points out, bio-medical science, like all forms of popular and esoteric knowledge, must use the imprecise medium of language to construct its systems of thought about the world, and this reliance in turn blurs the claims of 'facts' to be only things-in-themselves, which language simply describes. She writes,

> The nature of the relationship between language and reality is highly problematic; and *AIDS* is not merely an invented label, provided to us by science ... for a clear-cut disease entity caused by a virus. Rather, the very nature of AIDS is constructed through language and in particular through the discourses of medicine and science; this construction is 'true' or 'real' only in certain specific ways – for example insofar as it successfully guides research or facilitates clinical control over the illness. The name *AIDS* in part *constructs* the disease and helps make it intelligible. We cannot therefore look 'through' language to determine what AIDS 'really' is. Rather we must explore the site where such determinations *really* occur and intervene at the point where meaning is created: in language.
>
> (Treichler, 1988: 31)

This dependence of bio-medical science on language is significant because the metaphoric systems and narratives used to represent HIV/AIDS scientifically are what links these representations to the broader culture's ideas about AIDS. While bio-medicine understands its ideas about HIV/AIDS to be derived purely from the factual reality of the disease, the following analysis will investigate certain points of continuity between these ideas and more general discriminatory ideas about HIV/AIDS.

Explicit Discriminatory Language

In all the textbooks examined, the sections on AIDS epidemiology contained the most explicit discriminatory language. The reasons for this are complex but derive in the first instance from epidemiology's conceptual reliance on categories of people to explain infectious processes. Oppenheimer (1992), in his history of AIDS epidemiology, relates that early in the US epidemic the Center for Disease Control justified its nomination of homosexual men, Haitians and haemophiliacs as 'high-risk groups' for AIDS on the basis that 'classification of individuals is intrinsic to any epidemiological investigation' (Oppenheimer, 1992: 61). Other medical disciplines are less likely to display explicitly discriminatory language because they deal only with body parts or processes, but epidemiology deals with the more political question of the classification and social behaviour of populations.

While it may be arguable whether the act of nomination of any particular social group as a 'risk-group' is in itself an act of discrimination, we have restricted ourselves here to a description of instances where the textbooks' designations of these categories exceeded neutral terminology and take on a punitive colouring. So, for example, only two of the texts examined, Fauci and Lane in Wilson *et al.* (1991) and Wodak and Gold in Richmond and Wakefield (1989) used the term 'intravenous drug users' rather than 'intravenous drug abusers' or 'drug addicts' when discussing HIV transmission through needle sharing.

Gay men are not so uniformly described in discriminatory terms but there are nevertheless a number of punitive references. In Jawetz *et al.* (1991:579) the chapter about AIDS and lentiviruses refers a number of times to 'promiscuous' homosexual men. It states, for example, that 'promiscuous homosexual activity has been recognised as a major risk factor for acquisition of the disease'. It also makes an explicit distinction between homosexual men and injecting drug users and 'normal persons' in the following passage.

> Antibodies to HIV are found in almost all patients with clinical AIDS and in patients with ... conditions described as AIDS-related complex. Promiscuous homosexual men and intravenous drug abusers also have a high prevalence of antibodies. In contrast, antibodies are rare in normal individuals.
>
> (Jawetz *et al.*, 1991: 578)

While epidemiology understands the term 'promiscuity' as simply a quantitative designation, the equivalent of saying a 'high number of sexual partners', its use can be understood as discriminatory in so far as it is understood to deviate from a 'normal' number of sexual partners. This implicit normativity can also be seen in the tendency of some of the texts to foreground and sensationalize certain sexual practices as though they were typical of all gay sexuality. Masur, in the chapter entitled 'Infections in Homosexual Men' in Mandell *et al.* (1990), asserts, for example, that homosexual sex often leads to infection, due to rectal damage. This is because, he claims,

> Fisting, the practice of inserting a fist into the rectum, sometimes up to the elbow, is a commonly performed sex act, as is the insertion of bottles, bats and a wide variety of prosthetic devices.
>
> (Masur in Mandell *et al.*, 1990: 2281)

This characterization of gay sexual practice is misleading in at least three senses. First, it is not supported by empirical evidence. Only one per cent of the men interviewed for Project Sigma reported having 'fisting' style sex within the previous month (Davies *et al.*, 1993) and no data is available for the other practices described as 'common' by Masur. Second, it is misleading because, by associating HIV and other infections with such sensational practices, it tends to divert attention from the fact that HIV can be very successfully transmitted by any kind of sex which involves penile penetration, either anal or vaginal. Heterosexual missionary position marital sex is a much more efficient route of HIV transmission than penetration with a bottle. Third, such a characterization involves a failure to acknowledge that gay communities both invented safe sex and practise it on a wide scale.

These depictions of gay male sexuality as promiscuous and perverse, and the reliance on this characterization to explain the higher concentration of HIV positivity in this group, contribute strongly to the notion that gay men 'deserve' HIV infection, a notion that surfaces regularly in the discrimination literature. The idea that some people living with AIDS are guilty, that is deserving of illness and to be blamed for the spread of HIV, and some are innocent, appears in these textbooks also in relation to vertical transmission – HIV-positive women who bear HIV-positive infants. This assessment is evident in the way that the infant's infection is the focus of attention, while the mother is represented only as the source of infection. For example, the introduction to the AIDS section of Roitt's *Essential Immunology* states that in first-world countries,

> ... the majority of [AIDS] cases so far have occurred in male homosexuals with other groups at risk including intravenous drug abusers, haemophiliacs ... and infants of sexually promiscuous or drug-addicted mothers. None the less, the number of infected heterosexuals is steadily increasing.
>
> (Roitt, 1991: 245–6)

Another textbook, *Mechanisms of Microbial Disease* (Schaechter *et al.*, 1989), uses as its sole case study about HIV infection the example of a 19-year-old prostitute with terminal AIDS who gives birth to an HIV positive infant. The focus of the case is exclusively on the medical management of the infant, who dies of AIDS at four months.

In addition to instances of the punitive characterization of various social groups, several of these textbooks engage in what could be described as medical triumphalism, the elevation of bio-medical solutions to the spread of HIV above other social solutions. Where the question of the prevention of infection is raised, these textbooks give first place to medical technologies such as vaccines and anti-viral therapy, sometimes to the exclusion of educational considerations, or proven low technologies like condoms, alto-gether. One text for example claims that,

> it is unlikely that antiviral treatment will ever eradicate the virus in an

infected person. For this reason, an effective vaccine is the only foreseeable intervention to prevent HIV-1 transmission, infection and disease.'

(Clements in Mandell *et al.*, 1990: 1112)

More common than this complete dismissal of social measures is their relegation to a secondary position after vaccines and antivirals, despite the fact that at the time of writing no workable vaccine has been produced, nor an antiviral whose effectiveness extends beyond deferral of some symptoms for two-to-three years.

This medical triumphalism may not be immediately obvious as a kind of discrimination, until it is contrasted with a more socially aware perspective. By elevating vaccines and medical intervention as the most important, if only potential, form of prevention, these texts gloss over the work of prevention already done by various kinds of community education, often by precisely the groups of people punitively described in the same textbooks. Only one of the textbooks acknowledges this work and its effectiveness. Fauci and Lane in Wilson *et al.* (1991) begin the section on prevention in their chapter about AIDS with the statement 'Education, counselling and behaviour modification are the cornerstones of prevention of HIV infection', and argue their case on the grounds that these measures have been proved by the success of various gay communities in lowering the incidence of new infections.

> The incidence of new infections per year among homosexual and bisexual men in certain high-prevalence cities such as San Francisco has decreased dramatically from the early years of the epidemic. This has resulted, at least in part, from behavioural modifications regarding the number of sex partners and safe sexual practices. Several studies indicate that condom use decreases the risk of HIV transmission.

(Fauci and Lane in Wilson *et al.*,1991: 1410)

Significantly, this text is also the most careful in its avoidance of punitive language in the description of people living with AIDS. It seems plausible that the authors' acknowledgment of the contribution of gay men and other groups to prevention also informs their more positive evaluation of these groups, and their general refusal to imply culpability.

While most of the epidemiological treatments of HIV/AIDS in these textbooks resort to some punitive terminology, the sections dealing with the control of HIV infection in hospital settings are the reverse. Only three of the textbooks investigated this issue but all of them take a strong position regarding the very low risk of occupational HIV infection for health-care workers if appropriate measures are used, and the unethical nature of medical discrimination against HIV seropositive patients.

A chapter by Henderson entitled 'HIV-1 in the Health Care Setting', in Mandell *et al.* (1990) which provides the most thorough treatment of the question, notes that the initial reaction of health-care workers to AIDS patients in the hospital was conditioned by its apparent resemblance to Hepatitis B, which is considered more infectious than HIV. Henderson reviews the literature about percutaneous exposure to HIV-infected blood or body fluids in the hospital setting and concludes that risk of infection is very low, far too low to warrant discriminatory treatment of HIV-positive patients. He writes,

> When contrasted with the occupational risks all of us have been taking for years, this new risk provided by AIDS/HIV-1 infection does not seem to warrant the attention that it has received. When assessed in the appropriate context, decisions not to provide care to HIV-1 infected individuals seem incongruent.
>
> (Henderson in Mandell *et al.*, 1990: 2227)

In other words, the textbooks that deal with the issue take an interventionist anti-discrimination position on the question of the treatment of HIV-positive patients.

Implicit Discriminatory Discourse in Medical Texts

Having interrogated medical texts for explicit instances of discriminatory language, we will turn to the metaphoric systems that medicine uses to imagine the processes associated with HIV infection.

The masculinity of the immune system

HIV is understood to cause disease through an attack upon the body's immune system and the use of certain cells of the immune system to reproduce itself. This sounds straightforward, until the immune system is considered not as a simple and self-evident fact but as an *idea*. What is the immune system understood to be? All of the immunological texts consulted for this study begin with a statement like the following.

> The human organism, from the time of conception, must maintain its integrity in the face of a changing and often threatening environment. Our bodies have many physiological mechanisms that permit us to adjust to basic variables such as temperature, supply of food and water, and physical injury. In addition, we must defend ourselves

against invasion and colonisation by foreign organisms. This defence ability is called *immunity.*

(Sell, 1987: 3)

Again, this may seem straightforward enough, until we consider the organizing metaphor of the idea of immunity, that of defence against foreign invaders. In other words, the immune system is conceptualized as the body's defence force, its standing army, and infection is understood as a state of war. This conceptualization is general to immunology, as a number of commentators have demonstrated in surveys of the literature (Martin, 1990; Montgomery, 1991). The textbooks confirm the generality of this idea at a number of points. One states, for example:

> We are engaged in constant warfare with the microbes which surround us and the processes of mutation and evolution have tried to select micro-organisms which have evolved means of evading our defence mechanisms.
>
> (Roitt, 1991: 203)

If the immune system is a defence force, than its particular cells are, logically speaking, its troops, who seek out and kill the 'foreign invader' virus or bacterium. While as Martin (1990) and Montgomery (1991) point out, the implications of this logic are more easily seen in popular science literature than in technical medical literature, nevertheless, the textbooks clearly utilize this metaphor for the immune system cells in statements like the following.

> Functional studies have identified lymphocyte populations that serve as natural killer (NK) cells and antibody-dependent killer cells in the surveillance of certain tumours and virus infected cells. The NK cell is defined as an effector cell that has the capacity for spontaneous cytotoxicity toward various target cells and is not MHC restricted'.
>
> (Stites and Terr, 1991: 19)

'Killer' cells, which carry out 'surveillance' and which attack 'target' cells are clearly functioning according to a military model, as is the description of lymphocytes as 'recruited' when they encounter a specific antigen (University of Sydney Faculty of Medicine, 1992: 6). The T-lymphocyte system that HIV 'targets' is conceptualized as holding a command position in the immunological army, which is why HIV infection leads to a general disabling of the immune system.

> The relationship between the depletion of T4 lymphocytes and profound immunosuppression is clear. Since the T4 lymphocyte

subset is responsible for the induction and/or regulation of virtually the entire immune system, the selective defect in this subset results in global impairment of components of immunity that depend, at least in part, on inductive signals from the immune system.

(Fauci and Lane in Wilson *et al.*, 1991: 1404)

So if the immune system is conceptualized along military lines, in what way does this metaphoric system lend itself to HIV-related discrimination? One of the implications of this metaphor is the *masculinity* of the immune system. Again, this explicitly gendered understanding is more easily seen in popular immunology. Dwyer's (1988) popular immunology text *The Body at War*, for example, regularly refers to lymphocytes as 'he'. Martin (1990) notes that masculinity in the immune system is most pronounced in relation to the T cells, which are represented as technically advanced and well trained, and whose death or depletion is cause for anxiety, while the macrophage line of cells sometimes appear as the feminine 'housekeepers' of the immune system.

There are also certain points in the textbooks, however, where this masculinity becomes explicit, rather than implied by its militarized language. Roitt, for example, tends to use feminine or impotence images to talk about bodily weakness or failures of the immune system. At one point the text states, 'The spleen is a very effective blood filter removing *effete* red and white blood cells' (Roitt, 1991: 110). At another we find an analogy made between the process of anergy, where B cells can recognize and bind antigen but remain inactivated, with an 'ageing roué'.

These anergic cells could bind antigen to their surface receptors but could not be activated. Like the aging roue wistfully drinking in the visual attractions of some young belle, these tolerised lymphocytes could 'see' the antigen but lack the ability to do anything about it.

(Roitt, 1991: 186)

While such explicit examples of these equations between 'effeminacy' and immunological weakness are very few in the textbooks under discussion, they nevertheless point towards a general logic in immunology that represents the health and vigour of the immune system in masculine terms. This implicit masculinity may remain inconsequential for the representation of diseases that have no bearing on sexual difference, but in the case of HIV/AIDS, which is strongly associated with homosexuality, that is 'effeminate' or 'perverted' masculinity, it may lend itself to a scientifically rationalized homophobia.

This is so because just as homophobia is a discriminatory reaction to a perceived threat to 'normal' masculinity, so too can HIV infection be understood as a threat to the healthy normal masculinity of the immune system. HIV infection is understood to work through the genetic 'infiltration' of the T4 cells, an infiltration which 'disarms' these cells and renders them unable to coordinate the rest of the immune system. By inserting its genetic code into the existing code of the T4 cell, HIV effectively transforms the cell into a producer of more HIV. In other words, HIV 'perverts' the normal operation of the immune system, rendering what should be the body's 'defence force' into the site for the replication of virus.

In this way, the bio-medical representation of HIV infection can be said to double the potential for homophobia associated with HIV. A gay man who is HIV positive appears as both a social and an immunological threat to the idea of healthy masculinity.

HIV transmission and the idea of culpability

Unlike some other viruses and bacteria, HIV is understood to have very limited ability to survive outside the body or to transmit itself other than directly from body to body, and from cell to cell. In this sense it is understood to be a fragile virus, easily 'inactivated' by common household disinfectants within 10 minutes (Jawetz *et al.*, 1991). The term virulence is used in microbiology to measure the ability of an organism both to 'invade' the host's body and to spread within it.

> *Virulence* provides a quantitative measure of pathogenicity, or the likelihood of causing disease ... Virulence factors refer to the properties ... that enable a microorganism to establish itself on or within a host of a particular species and enhance its potential to cause disease.
>
> (Relman and Falkow in Mandell *et al.*, 1990: 25)

The first factor in determining virulence is necessarily the pathogen's ability to gain access to its host in sufficient numbers.

> Gaining access to a potential host requires that the microorganism not only make contact with an appropriate surface but also then reach its unique niche or micro-environment on or within the host. This requirement is not trivial. Some pathogens must survive for varying lengths of time in the external environment. Others have evolved an effective and suitable means of transmission.
>
> (Relman and Falkow in Mandell *et al.*, 1990: 26)

Because HIV is a fragile virus, it must transmit itself to a new host contained within certain infected cells of its existing host, without any detours through the external environment.

29

> HIV enters the host contained within infected cells, e.g. macrophages,
> lymphocytes or spermatozoa. Such cells are deposited in tissues and
> enter the body either through microabrasions on the surface of
> mucous membranes or through penetration of intact skin with a
> needle.
>
> (Meissner and Coffin in Schaechter *et al.*, 1989: 442)

Once HIV has established itself within a host, however, infection continues for
the lifetime of the host.

> The biology of human retroviruses is such that once the host has been
> infected, there is permanent integration of viral material in the form
> of proviral genome in the [DNA] of the host target cells. This provirus
> is capable of replication and production of new virions. From an
> epidemiologic point of view, therefore, a person with evidence of
> prior infection ... must be considered permanently infected and
> potentially infectious to others.
>
> (Groopman in Wyngaarden and Smith, 1988:1799)

The HIV-positive person with no symptoms is thus understood as an 'asymptomatic carrier', a person whose immune system has been given over to the
incubation of the virus, but who displays no outward signs of infection. To be
the 'carrier' of a fragile virus that cannot live outside the body implies that the
HIV-positive person is the virus's means of mobility. Furthermore, the HIV-
positive person must 'act' in order to transmit virus. They must have sexual
relations, or share a syringe, or give birth or breastfeed an infant, because only
direct exchange of certain body fluids provides the virus with the right kind
of pathway into another body.

In other words, human agency is understood to be implicated in the
'microbial virulence' of the HIV, an understanding implied by terms like
'carrier' for a person living with AIDS. It is this understanding, we think, that
appears in some of the more lurid statements about gay sexual practices cited
in the previous section, and which underpins the notion that some categories
of the HIV-positive person, particularly gay men and injecting drug users, are
both undeserving of sympathy and responsible for the epidemic.

The HIV-positive person as viral representative

The understanding of the HIV-positive person as a 'carrier' of virus is an
extension of the particular bio-medical notion of HIV's 'microbial virulence',
but it is also an expression of the idea that the identity of the person infected
with HIV is colonized by the virus. This idea of identity colonization arises

from two prior medical conceptualizations. The first of these is the idea that the immune system simultaneously constitutes and defends the person's biological identity. This can be seen in some statements made in the textbooks. For example, Roitt refers to the immune system as the means by which the body defends itself against genetic colonization.

> We live in a potentially hostile world filled with a bewildering array of infectious agents of diverse shape, size, composition and subversive character which would happily use us as rich sanctuaries for propagating their 'selfish genes' had we not developed a series of defence mechanisms at least their equal in effectiveness and ingenuity ... It is these defence mechanisms which can establish a state of immunity against infection.
>
> (Roitt, 1991: 1)

The immune system is understood to defend against such microbial colonization through its ability to distinguish 'self'' from 'non-self' and to attack 'non-self' (Sell, 1987: 9). On this model then, all forms of infection count as a compromise of the distinction between 'self' and 'non-self'.

This idea of compromise is more pronounced in the case of viral infection than in the case of bacterial infection because viruses are understood to reproduce through the use of the host cell's reproductive apparatus. This is the second strand of the idea of HIV infection as colonization of identity. HIV, like all viruses, comprises little more than its own genetic material, which overrides the host cell genome and 'instructs' the host cell to make virus. This idea of genetic 'reprogramming' of the cell carries more consequences for the bio-medical notion of organism identity because an organism's genes are considered to be effectively its repository of identity, its site of biological 'instructions' for proper self-replication. As Diprose and Vasseleau note, the genetic code is understood in current bio-medical science to be completely determining of the organism.

> Biomedical science has thus developed a model of the body as ... a simplistic text the form of which is derived from the message, the genetic code ... DNA [is] the repeated sub-unit or genetic code. The genetic instructions are 'copied' by the duplication of DNA; 'transcribed' into the alphabet of the unstable messenger RNA; and 'translated' by stable forms of RNA from four-letter codes into twenty-letter coding of proteins. These proteins are responsible for cell structure, and the relations between cells give us the morphology of the whole.
>
> (Diprose and Vasseleau, 1991: 150–151)

So, while all infection counts as a compromise of the biological 'self', viral infection is more of a compromise, and infection with HIV is still more of a compromise. HIV represents the current pinnacle of such a notion because it is understood to attack the body's cells that are most heavily implicated in the protection of biological identity, the T4-cells, and because it effects the most profound kind of transformation in these cells' genome. The retroviruses, the family of viruses to which the HIV belongs, are characterized by their ability to integrate their genetic material directly into the DNA of the host cell and to remain latent for long periods of time.

> [A] salient feature of retroviruses is the integration of the DNA intermediate into the host cell DNA. Consequently, infections can be lifelong, and the virus may remain 'hidden' (unexpressed or non-replicative) in cells for very long periods. This may contribute to the long intervals (sometimes many years) between the time of infection and disease induction.
>
> (Gallo in Wyngaarden and Smith, 1988: 1794)

This genetic integration means that the T4 cells so colonized begin to act as sites for the virus to replicate itself, leading to both depletion in the overall number of T4 cells and to their malfunctioning. The virus now effectively occupies the position at the top of the immunological hierarchy and so the new genetic information it provides to the T4 cell acts as a 'disinformation' programme for many of the central processes of the immune system. In addition to the eventual cytopathic effect of HIV infection for the individual T4 cell, a number of qualitative abnormalities in other aspects of the immune response are described in the textbooks, including: selective deficiency of cutaneous hypersensitivity responses; failure of T4 cells from AIDS patients to proliferate in response to soluble antigen *in vitro*; absence of an *in vivo* response to tetanus toxoid antigen in HIV-positive persons with a normal number of circulating T4 cells; impaired cytotoxic responses, for example depressed response against cytomegalovirus and influenza; impairment of antigen-specific and non-specific B cell responses (e.g. poor response to immunization, erratic immunoglobulin production); impaired Natural Killer cell surveillance.

These transformations in the functioning of the immune system mean that the HIV-positive person's immune system effectively loses what is understood to be its primary ability and *raison d'etre*; it can no longer distinguish self from non-self, becoming what is known as 'immunocompromised'.

> The disease state called acquired immunodeficiency syndrome (AIDS) is at the terminal stage ... when the infected host can no longer control opportunistic organisms or malignancies that rarely

cause illness in immunocompetent individuals. In persons infected with HIV, the sequential decline and ablation of cell-mediated immunity result in diverse manifestations of opportunistic disease.

(Chaisson and Volberding in Mandell *et al.*, 1990: 1059)

In other words, because the immune system is understood to be constitutive of 'biological identity', and because HIV infection is understood as an annexation of this system for the purposes of the virus, the HIV-positive person's 'biological identity' becomes almost synonymous with the virus.

Conclusions

The metaphoric systems we have traced here remain implicit in medical discourse about HIV and are not necessarily mobilized in discriminatory practice in medical settings. Yet they form a kind of repository of unconscious images that inform the medical imagination about HIV/AIDS and which contribute, we argue, to general tendencies among health-care workers towards moralistic and judgemental positions in relation to people living with AIDS.

Our study thus has serious implications for the way that HIV-related discrimination, and strategies to overcome it, have been conceptualized. It points towards the necessity to subject not only medical practice but also medical knowledge to critical scrutiny, in the formulation of such strategies. It also indicates the need to encourage a critical attitude towards medical knowledge on the part of health-care students, in the same way that a critical position is developed in humanities and social science teaching practice. Furthermore, it throws into question the tendency of some AIDS activist groups to take the usefulness and factual simplicity of medical knowledge for granted, a tendency which this study indicates may work against the interests of people living with AIDS.

References

BOLTON, R. (1992) 'AIDS and Promiscuity', *Medical Anthropology*, 14, 144–223.

DAVIES, P.M., HICKSON, F.C.I., WEATHERBURN, P. and HUNT, A.J. (1993) *Sex, Gay Men and AIDS*, London: Taylor & Francis.

DIPROSE R. and VASSELEAU, C. (1991) 'Animation – AIDS and science/fiction', in CHOLODENKO, A. (Ed.) *The Illusion of Life. Essays on Animation*, Sydney: Power Publications.

DWYER, J. (1988) *THE BODY AT WAR: THE STORY OF OUR IMMUNE SYSTEM*, SYDNEY: ALLEN AND UNWIN.

EPSTEIN, S. (1988) 'Moral contagion and the medicalisation of gay identity: AIDS in historical perspective', *Research in Law, Deviance and Social Control*, **9**, 3–36.

FLECK, L. (1979) *Genesis and Development of a Scientific Fact*, translated by Fred Bradley and Thaddeus Trenn, Chicago: University of Chicago Press.

GOSTIN, L. (1992) 'The AIDS Litigation Project: A National Review of Court and Human Rights Decisions on Discrimination', in Fee, E. and Fox, D. (Eds) *AIDS: the Making of a Chronic Disease*, Berkeley, University of California Press.

JAWETZ, E., MELNICK, J., ADELBERG E. *et al.* (1991) *Medical Microbiology*, nineteenth edition, London: Prentice-Hall.

MANDELL, G., DOUGLAS, R.G., and BENNETT, J. (1990) (Eds) *Principles and Practice of Infectious Diseases*, vols I and II, third edition, New York: Churchill Livingstone.

MARTIN E. (1990) 'Towards an anthropology of immunology: The body as nation state', *Medical Anthropology Quarterly*, **4**(4), 410–426.

MONTGOMERY, S. (1991) 'Codes and combat in bio-medical discourse', *Science as Culture*, **2**, 341–391.

NEW SOUTH WALES ANTI-DISCRIMINATION BOARD (1992) 'Discrimination – The Other Epidemic', report of the Inquiry into HIV and AIDS Related Discrimination.

OPPENHEIMER, G. (1992) 'Causes, cases, and cohorts: The role of epidemiology in the historical construction of AIDS', in FEE, E. AND FOX, D. (Eds) *AIDS: the Making of a Chronic Disease*, Berkeley, University of California Press.

PATTON, C. (1990) *Inventing AIDS*, New York: Routledge.

RICHMOND, R. and WAKEFIELD D. (Eds) (1989) *AIDS and Other Sexually Transmitted Diseases*, Sydney: Harcourt Brace Jovanovich.

ROITT, I. (1991) *Essential Immunology*, seventh edition, Oxford: Blackwell Scientific Publications.

SCHAECHTER, M., MEDOFF, G. and SCHLESSINGER, D. (Eds) (1989) *Mechanisms of Microbial Disease*, Baltimore: Williams and Wilkins.

SELL, S. (1987) *Basic Immunology. Immune Mechanisms in Health and Disease*, London: Elsevier.

STITES, D. and TERR A. (Eds) (1991) *Basic and Clinical Immunology*, London: Prentice-Hall.

TREICHLER, P. (1988) 'AIDS, homophobia and biomedical discourse: An epidemic of signification', in CRIMP, D. (Ed.) *AIDS: Cultural Analysis, Cultural Activism*, Cambridge, MA: Massachusetts Institute of Technology Press.

UNIVERSITY OF SYDNEY (1992) Faculty of Medicine, Immunology Notes, Med III 1992.

WILSON, J., BRAUNWALD, E., ISSELBACHER, K. *et al.* (Eds) (1991) *Harrison's Principles of Internal Medicine*, vols I and II, twelfth edition, New York: McGraw-Hill.

WYNGAARDEN, J. and SMITH, L. (Eds) (1988) *Cecil Textbook of Medicine*, vols I and II, eighteenth edition, Philadelphia: W.B. Saunders.

Chapter 3

Travel, Sexual Behaviour and Gay Men

Stephen Clift and John Wilkins

From the early years of the HIV/AIDS epidemic, it was apparent that international travel – for business and for pleasure – played a necessary though not sufficient role in the geographic and social diffusion of HIV infection (Conway *et al.*, 1990; Gould, 1993; Hawkes, 1992; Hawkes and Hart, 1993). HIV is transmitted from person to person primarily by unprotected penetrative sex or through sharing of injecting equipment. Consequently, its initial emergence within the resident populations of regions, countries and districts previously unaffected, must have been due to contact with individuals from 'elsewhere'; either by uninfected individuals travelling away from home to areas where HIV infection was present, or through contact with HIV-infected persons visiting an area initially free from infection. As Conway, Gillies and Slack (1990) note, the majority of the early cases of AIDS reported in Denmark, Italy, Germany and the United Kingdom, were among 'men who had had sexual contacts with men who lived in the United States'. Equally, the crucial significance of travel in the early stages of the development of the epidemic in the USA, is graphically illustrated by Gould's (1993) account of the epidemiological work that led to the identification of the so-called 'Patient Zero':

> The sexual contacts of 40 men who had converted to AIDS were carefully traced (. . .), and led to the probable identification of Patient Zero, later identified as an airline steward with international connections. Even within the United States the trail of structuring connections led from Los Angeles, to New York, to San Francisco, and five other states, and most of the men reported large numbers of sexual partners. (. . .) Whether Patient Zero was the initiator of the pandemic in the United States will never be known with certainty, and in any event it is of little importance since at a global scale airline travel

virtually guarantees rapid transmission (...) It is reasonable to assume that he was infected in the early seventies (...) and then spread the virus to perhaps scores or even hundreds of partners.

(p. 38)

As the HIV/AIDS epidemic has developed, few regions in the world have remained free of cases of infection and a complex spatial and socio-cultural 'geography' of many overlapping epidemics has evolved with higher incidence levels in some physical locations and social 'spaces', and lower incidences in others (see e.g. Anderson, 1993; Mertens *et al.*, 1994). There is some evidence which counters the view that travel is associated with changes in sexual behaviour (Mårdh, 1994) and enhanced risk of HIV infection (Garland *et al.*, 1993). However, the mobility of non-infected and infected individuals (Cohn *et al.*, 1994) both within and across national boundaries, combined with behaviour that allows for HIV transmission, may continue to be a significant factor influencing the evolving dynamics of the global pandemic. Lewis and Bailey (1993), for example, consider the potential impact of international mobility on the prevalence of HIV/AIDS in the Pacific Islands, currently an area of low incidence:

> Although to date relatively few cases of AIDS have been diagnosed in the Pacific Islands, the relationship between AIDS and population movement has important implications for the region. The economies of many of these states are heavily tourism-dependent. For some of the islands states there is also considerable circular migration, particularly between the home islands and New Zealand, Hawaii and the mainland United States. There is also mobility between and within the islands, and some movement between the Pacific Islands and neighbouring Asian nations.

(p. 159)

The fact that sexual transmission of HIV requires close physical contact between infected and uninfected individuals provides the apparent rationale for Draconian public health measures, such as quarantine, introduced by a small number of countries (e.g. Cuba and Bangladesh, see Gould, 1993) and for the imposition of entry restrictions on HIV-infected persons introduced by rather more (see Alcorn, 1995, for details). Nevertheless, it is more widely accepted internationally that freedom of movement not only constitutes a fundamental human right (Chang-Muy, 1993) but is, moreover, an essential factor in the construction and operation of transnational free-market economies. Thus, the fight against HIV/AIDS has relied primarily on new public health strategies of social and educational interventions to encourage modifications of lifestyle, reductions of risky behaviour and the strengthening of personal and community responsibility for health – within social and cultural contexts that allow substantial numbers of people considerable freedom of movement. A further factor which needs to be considered is that travel to new destinations may provide enhanced opportunities for socio-sexual interactions which may not be available, or taken advantage of, in the home environment. As the NAM *AIDS Reference Manual* (Alcorn, 1995) notes:

> There is also a tendency for people to take sexual opportunities whilst abroad which would be denied to them at home. A classic example is the way in which visitors to London feel able to participate in the gay scene and have sex with men which would be unthinkable in their home towns, or male travellers having sex with prostitutes whilst abroad.
>
> (p. 45)

In addition, in the case of holidays, individuals are 'at leisure' and may actively seek the pleasure and excitement of new sexual encounters under the influence of a holiday mood enhanced sometimes by increased alcohol consumption and recreational drug use (see Clark and Clift, 1995; Ford and Eiser, 1995; Gillies and Slack, 1995; for discussions of holidays as a context for sex).

Concern regarding the continuing significance of all kinds of mobility in relation to HIV/AIDS, provides the rationale for HIV/AIDS prevention efforts targeted towards migrants, travellers and holiday-makers, whether on a European scale (the European Project 'AIDS and Mobility', see Bröring, 1995; and the Europe against AIDS – Summer Campaign), a national level (see Stears, 1995 for an account of the UK Department of Health's 'Travelsafe' campaign) or within localities (see Ford *et al.*, 1995; Stears, 1995). Such campaigns may be inherently problematic, however, in serving to reinforce myths that the danger of HIV infection resides away from home in certain dangerous locations (Carter, 1994) or is linked with the 'cultural other' (Schiller *et al.*, 1994). Wellings (1994) provides an instructive account of the issues that HIV/AIDS prevention campaigns targeted at travellers have had to consider, and examples where mistakes have been made:

> Interventions had to be designed which gave no hint of xenophobia, nor of making the assumption that people in other countries were riskier than people at home, i.e., that risk was inherent in the behaviour of the traveller and not in the people of the country being visited. An instance in which this was not achieved is (...) to be found in Sweden, where an advertisement showing a gay bar in Copenhagen came under fire from the Danes, and a picture of the Eiffel Tower [constructed from condom packets and accompanied with the slogan

'Oh-la-la'] brought injured criticism from the French Embassy.

(p. S26)

Such material may also serve to strengthen prejudices towards marginalized groups and to reinforce a sense of the irrelevance of HIV/AIDS among those as yet not directly affected by it. There is a possibility, therefore, that a chapter such as this, which aims to consider recent evidence relating to travel, sexual behaviour and gay men, may be seen as irrelevant to the urgent task of HIV prevention with gay men who continue to be at risk in their home environ- ments, or worse, as positively harmful in serving only to strengthen a formidable and dangerous amalgam of homo- and xeno-phobia. We would disassociate ourselves immediately from any such implications or use of the material we intend to consider below, and argue instead that a serious examination of the travel/tourist behaviour of gay men, and the extent to which sexual activity in the context of travel either involves or enhances risks of HIV infection among gay men, is warranted, and may have value in relation to the planning and targeting of effective intervention strategies. In this regard, it is interesting to note that the London-based organization *Gay Men Fighting AIDS* has recently launched a campaign entitled 'Cumming Away' in association with 'Shades', a specialist gay tour operator, to remind gay men of the need to practice safer sex while on holiday (GMFA, 1994; see also *Steam* magazine, February 1995).

The aim of this chapter is to provide a critical review of the surprisingly sparse and disparate research literature that addresses the sexual behaviour and sexual health risks of gay men in the context of international travel and tourism. Before examining such research studies, however, it is of interest to consider travel and tourism among gay men, as such. This is an interesting topic in its own right quite apart from the specific sexual health dimensions highlighted so far in this discussion – not only with respect to the extent, nature and meaning of travel and tourism in the context of gay cultures and personal lifestyles, but also in terms of the economics, planning and management of gay tourist services, the marketing of gay tourist products, the sociological and psychological dimen- sions of the gay tourist experience and not least, the impact of gay tourism on the host communities resident in mass tourism destinations. There is remarkably little serious writing on gay travel and tourism. This is indicated by the lack of any reference to gay men as tourists in the recently published volume *Tourism: The State of the Art* (Seaton, 1994) and the fact that enquiries to the 'Centre des Hautes Etudes Touristiques', a major tourism research resource centre in Aix- en-Provence, France, provided no information on existing studies. Computer assisted searches of the social science and psychological literature revealed only a few historical studies of gay travel, which are of minor significance in relation to an understanding of contemporary patterns of gay travel (e.g. Austen, 1983; Poirier, 1993) or strangely obscure (e.g. Bleys, 1993).

Gay Men, Travel and Tourism

One historical source that is of some interest, however, is Aldrich's (1993) account of the association between the Mediterranean and 'homoeroticism' as seen through the works of northern European writers, artists, art critics and photographers. According to Aldrich, the Mediterranean was 'the central theme in homoerotic writing and art from the 1750s to the 1950s' and this encouraged generations of homosexual men, from less hospitable northern European countries to travel south, in search of sexual expression and a sense of identity. 'Those with sexual desires which contravene the socially accepted norms of their countries', he argues, 'have often become expatriates, figuratively by searching for hospitable cultures for study and emulation and in actual fact as they travel overseas for holidays or go into exile.'

Such journeying by homosexual men to southern climes, and the image of the homoerotic south, generated by numerous artists and writers, was especially significant from the late eighteenth to the mid-nineteenth centuries. During the last decades of the last century and the early years of this, however, 'the myth of the homoerotic Mediterranean began to lose its potency', and eventually with the development of 'gay liberation' from the late 1960s onwards, 'a period of militant campaigns for gay rights' fostered behaviours and attitudes which, in Aldrich's view, departed markedly from 'the Mediterranean fantasy'. The current association between the Mediterranean and gay men is summed up by Aldrich in the following terms:

> The Mediterranean has remained a favoured destination of gay tourists, who went to Mykonos in the 1960s and now travel to Ibiza and Sitges, where the beach and the Mediterranean town-squares provided the backgrounds for gay bars and discos. Visits to the sites preferred by earlier generations of homosexuals are now only part and parcel of the new grand tour of travellers or represent a specifically gay pilgrimage. (...) A gay travel guide lists addresses for the 'Antinous' massage parlour or the 'Mykonos' sauna in northern cities; these are the reminders, but little more, of a powerful cultural legacy that is part of gay history. A new culture, that of gay urban America, triumphed over the old Mediterranean in the 1970s, although it has lately been endangered by AIDS. New icons – the 'disco queen', the macho male, the respectable and openly gay middle-class homosexual, the 'gender-fuck' androgyne, the young 'queer' activist – replaced the Mediterranean ephebe and the dance music of discos has taken the place of the classical poetry and mythology dear to the homosexuals of the nineteenth century.
>
> (p. 145)

For the post-war period, no systematic attempt has yet been made to document the development and scale of travel/tourism undertaken by gay men. Such a survey would provide an interesting complementary volume to Aldrich's scholarly historical review. It is obvious, however, that tourism among gay men must have developed rapidly from the late 1950s onwards in line with general trends in the scale of international travel and tourism and that currently, the level of international travel/tourism among gay men is substantial. Tourism Industry Intelligence (TII, 1994), for instance, suggests that an 'estimated 5 million to 25 million gay men and lesbians buy more than $10 billion worth of travel every year.'

Reference to publications such as *Spartacus* (an international gay guide published in Berlin) offers the gay traveller/tourist detailed information on the 'attractions' of destinations worldwide. The length of the entries in the *Spartacus* guide, provides a clear indication of those destinations that are likely to be particularly attractive to gay men from other countries. The entries are organized under a number of headings (e.g. bars, clubs, hotels, sex shops, escort agencies, saunas, information services, social centres and HIV/AIDS organizations), which reflect the development of gay businesses along side the establishment of venues and settings where consensual sex or sex for money takes place. As Table 3.1 suggests, the cities with the most developed gay commercial infrastructures are to be found in northern Europe and the USA.

Table 3.1 Ten 'important gay cities' with the largest entries identified in the 1994/95 Spartacus Guide

Country	Cities	Number of pages
France	Paris	38
Germany	Berlin	32
	Hamburg	18
	Cologne	14
	Munich	17
	Frankfurt	12
Netherlands	Amsterdam	23
United States	Los Angeles	10
	New York City	15
	San Francisco	16

Further details of holiday destinations attracting gay tourists can be found in brochures produced by specialist tour companies catering for gay men, and such businesses would undoubtedly have a wealth of experience of gay men as travellers. The British tour company 'Uranian Travel', for example, says of itself:

We have been organising gay holidays for more than 18 years so you can book with confidence and complete peace of mind. Uranian

Travel is Europe's largest gay tour operator and offers a comprehensive travel service under the reliable umbrella of Infocus Leisure Services Limited. All the staff employed by Uranian Travel are gay and naturally with our experience over the years we have great insight into the travel requirements of our clients and understand what you require from your holiday.

(The Uranian Experience brochure, 1995: 2)

The destinations included in the 1995 brochure are: Sitges, Ibiza, Playa del Ingles, Palma and Mykonos, together with city breaks to Amsterdam and Paris, and 'RSVP Cruises' in the Caribbean, the Mexican Riviera and off the coast of California. The following quotation from the entry on Sitges reflects the tenor of the brochure and clearly suggests that the opportunity for sexual encounters is one of the things that gay men 'require' from a holiday:

Sip a glass of local wine in a pavement cafe and let the Spanish way of life embrace you while you decide your next move. There are plenty of gay bars and discos to explore for those close encounters of the romantic kind. After a leisurely breakfast ease yourself into the day, flop on the beach and spend a few languorous moments contemplating your navel or somebody else's. A dip in the sea will refresh body and soul turning your mind towards another night of pleasure.

(p. 4)

Travel features in the gay press provide a more discerning perspective on popular gay destinations and in the process provide interesting insights into patterns of gay travel, the attractions of different destinations and the ways in which destinations have changed over time. Recent travel features in British gay/lesbian magazines such as *Attitude, Gay Times* and *Phase* have focused on popular European destinations (e.g. Ibiza and Paris), destinations further afield equally attractive to the gay traveller, (e.g. San Francisco and Sydney), together with destinations off the beaten gay track (e.g. Iceland and Vietnam). Major international gay events in 1994 that attracted thousands of overseas visitors – the celebrations of the 25th anniversary of the Stonewall riots and the Gay Games in New York – have also been featured in *Gay Times* (August 1994) and *Phase* (August/September 1994). A systematic analysis of travel features in the gay press over time could provide a valuable starting point for a serious study of the development and character of gay tourism, but here two examples must suffice.

In the feature on Ibiza in *Gay Times*, Richard Smith (1994) informs us that gay men formed the second wave of tourists who began to be attracted to the island in the late 1970s, after the visits by groups of hippies in the 1960s. And today 'Ibiza is only rivalled by Sitges as *the* European gay resort'. However:

> Ibiza may be as gay as a pink poodle in hot pants, but the majority of gay visitors are of a more mature vintage – thirty and fortysomethings who come back every year – and much of the gay bar scene is set up to cater for them.
>
> (p. 96)

As for the 'romance', 'pleasure' and 'contemplating somebody else's navel' that was promised in the Uranian Travel brochure, Smith's account suggests that the last of these three is more readily on offer than the first and second:

> There aren't many touristy things to do in Ibiza. Which suits me just fine. Days are invariably spent on the beach. Nudity's the norm on all beaches outside the towns, and on the big gay beach of Es Cavellet most of the people taking their clothes off are, hallelujah, the sort of boys you want to see butt naked. With its mixture of pan-European queens (mainly English and German) and a few Americans, the place is as uninhibited as a kiddies' playground. There's also some action in the bushes and dunes just behind the beach but, sadly, the spunk was hardly forming its own course down to the sea when I went.
>
> (p. 98)

Looking beyond the Mediterranean to the Antipodes, Kerry Bashford (1995) in a fascinating feature in *Attitude* magazine on the Sydney Mardi Gras claims that Sydney 'has always been the gay capital of the southern hemisphere'. What is especially interesting, in the context of the present discussion, is that the Mardi Gras has become a major attraction to international tourists, with 'Sydney during February becoming the essential destination for the intrepid queer'. And since 'Sydney's annual queerfest is now the biggest event of its kind in the world' visitors add 'millions of dollars to the coffers of Australia's tourist industry'.

A compilation of gay travel writing is brought together by American authors Gelder and Brandt (1992) in their companion for the gay and lesbian traveller – *Are You Two . . . Together? A Gay and Lesbian Guide to Europe*. The book aims to address the scarcity of 'gay travel writing', avoid the single-minded focus of so many gay guidebooks on bars and cruising and provide the traveller with insights into local gay culture and history. The book is also practical and provides information for gay and lesbian travellers on the best places to stay and eat to avoid 'the specter of homophobia', and on 'where to find each other – including those of us who aren't necessarily on the prowl for a trick or a lover'. Gay men and lesbians, they suggest, may be 'natural travellers', not only because they are more likely to have a higher disposable income, or because they need more often to get away from 'the literal straightjacket of the workaday closet', but also because 'the outsider perspective of the traveler is a second skin to us'. But gay travellers abroad are fortunate in having 'a resource other visitors don't:

> ... a built-in international community of our own. Long before 1992, gay Europeans were sharing a culture, which is your culture too. Walk into a gay bar or center in any country, and you stand a good chance of walking out with new friends (...) You may be a foreigner, but you won't be a stranger.

> (p. xvi)

Perhaps the only academic account of contemporary gay tourism yet produced is Luongo and Holcomb's (1995) paper on 'Geographical aspects of gay tourism in the USA' in which they describe the spatial pattern of gay tourism, discuss its economic significance and provide examples of recent gay tourist events. Such forces as legislation against gay men/lesbians and social prejudice from heterosexuals, coupled with the wish to meet like-minded people, and to pursue opportunities for sex and friendship have encouraged 'the spatial concentration or specialization of gay tourist destinations' in the USA. The gay tourism market is 'strong, large and growing' since gay male couples, in particular, are likely to have a high joint earning power and are unlikely to have children. As a result their disposable income will be substantially higher than heterosexual couples of comparable occupational status. Consequently, they claim, 'gay couples average 4.5 trips a year compared to the straight average of one'. A recent issue of Tourism Intelligence reinforces these points (TII, 1994).

Specific events attracting gay and lesbian visitors provide clear evidence of the economic significance of gay tourism. The Gay and Lesbian March on Washington (April 1993), for instance, may have attracted up to one million visitors to the city and the event had a significant impact on the capital's hotels and transportation networks. Increased revenue to the city due directly to the March is estimated to be $177 million. The Gay Games IV, held in New York City in June 1994 attracted nearly 11,000 athletes from 44 countries. This, claims Luongo and Holcomb, made it 'the largest multi-sport event in world history'. The exact revenues from the games are not known, but estimates have put them at $378 million. The week of the games also saw major celebrations of the 25th anniversary of the Stonewall riots, including 'the largest educational exhibit on gays and lesbians ever held in United States' at the main branch of the New York Public Library, a celebratory concert at Carnegie Hall and an Anniversary parade:

> As a cumulative total, over one million gays and lesbians came in to New York City through the week, making it the largest movement of homosexuals in world history. Over 500 thousand came in for the

Anniversary parade alone on Sunday the 26th.

(p. 9)

This brief survey of sources on gay travel and tourism hardly begins to address the many dimensions of gay travel and tourism as a cultural and commercial phenomenon, but it does provide some indication of the major parameters of scale and spatialization. Further research is needed to explore the personal travel motivations of gay men, the destinations they choose and their experiences while travelling and on holiday abroad.

Travel, Sexual Behaviour and Gay Men

To date, the topic of travel and sexual activity among gay men does not appear to have been addressed by major groups of researchers concerned with gay men and AIDS. Thus, a recent paper on 'men who have sex with men' arising out of the EC concerted action on the assessment of AIDS/HIV prevention strategies, makes no mention of travel and tourism (Pollak *et al.*, 1994); travel as an issue was not addressed in the WHO/GPA 'Homosexual Response Studies' conducted in seven countries (Coxon, 1992); and a major overview of research and prevention initiatives for gay men (King, 1993) makes no reference to travel and tourism. This lack of attention may reflect the political sensitivities noted in the introduction, judgements that risks in the context of travel are minor compared with those 'at home' and raise no particular or special issues of interest, or research priorities focused on proximal psychological and inter-personal factors affecting patterns of sexual activity and condom use. The consequence is that there are surprisingly few research studies concerned with gay men, travel and sexual behaviour, and those that do exist are so diverse in terms of context, methodology, sampling, information gathered and forms of analysis employed, that generalizations are difficult to formulate. In the following sections, attention is focused on those investigations which have reported data on patterns of travel and sexual behaviour among 'gay' men. The inverted commas are necessary because none of the projects reviewed seriously addressed the issue of personal identity and the extent of 'gay identification' among the men studied. The review looks first at research conducted in tourist destinations with men who are sexually active while there, and then at studies conducted in clinic settings subsequent to travel abroad.

Wilke and Kleiber (1992) report an investigation of homosexual men visiting Thailand which addressed four questions: which men visited Thailand as 'sex tourists'; why do homosexual men engage in sex on holiday; what sexual activities do they practice, and how often are condoms used? Ninety-four German male tourists who had had sex with Thai men were interviewed in Pattaya, a centre for sex tourism, during January/February 1992. The men interviewed were aged from 20 to 60 and above, with relatively more in the 40–49 and 50–59 age groups when compared with the general German male population. Less than 20 per cent were visiting Thailand for the first time and 'many of them visited the country frequently for the purpose of having sex with Thai men/boys'. On average, they reported having had sex with eight Thai men/boys during their stay (with a median of four) and 41 per cent of the tourist reported having sex with five or more men/boys. The length of contact was surprisingly variable: 20 per cent of men reported being with their last partner for up to two hours, while 40 per cent reported being with their last partner for 'several days'.

A wide range of sexual practices were apparent with active and passive fellatio reported by approximately 75 per cent of men and active and passive rimming (oral-anal contact) reported by between 20 per cent and 30 per cent. A marked difference was apparent for receptive and active anal intercourse, however, with just under 30 per cent of men reporting receptive anal intercourse compared with just under 50 per cent reporting active inter-course. In relation to insertive intercourse, 17 per cent of men 'never' used a condom, 15 per cent 'sometimes' used one and 68 per cent 'always' used one. Condom use was reported to be more consistent during receptive intercourse – with 82 per cent of men always using them. Such data need to be interpreted cautiously, however, since there is likely to be strong social desirability factor affecting the information given.

Data on numbers of sex partners 'at home' suggested that in a significant proportion of cases the German tourists had not been sexually active during the previous year. Thus, 35 per cent of men had not had a steady partner over that time and 35 per cent had not had a 'spontaneous' sexual partner. For another sizeable group, however, their pattern of sexual behaviour while on holiday appeared to be an extension of their usual lifestyle rather than behaviour specific to the holiday context. Thus, 27.5 per cent of men had had two or more 'steady' partners in the last year; 32 per cent had had sex with a male prostitute and 48.5 per cent of men had had two or more 'spontaneous' sexual partners over the same period.

The German tourists were also asked about other holiday destinations and sexual activity over the previous five years. The results showed clearly that sexual activity on holiday was highly prevalent across four continents. Thus, out of 28 men having a holiday in Asia during the past 5 years, 71 per cent reported sexual intercourse; out of 18 visiting Africa, 83 per cent reported sexual activity; out of 18 visiting the USA/Canada, 89 per cent reported sex and of 19 visiting Latin America, 47 per cent reported sex.

In discussing these findings, Wilke and Kleiber acknowledge that their sample is probably unrepresentative of homosexual travellers in general since they were concerned with gay men who paid for sexual contact with Thai men. The decision to focus on this group was motivated by the greater ease of contacting tourists in 'locations sought out mainly by male prostitutes and their customers'. It is clear from the results that substantial levels of risk behaviour were found. Almost a third of homosexual men reporting insertive intercourse did not use condoms consistently, and just over 40 per cent of men in the sample reported sex with five or more Thai boys/men. Reported levels of self-protection during receptive intercourse were higher suggesting either that a proportion of German gay men saw little or no risk to themselves during active insertive penetration or had little regard for the welfare of their Thai partners.

No data are reported on the proportion of gay men who visited Thailand specifically to have sex with young boys, but this was clearly a significant aspect of some of the men's behaviour. As the authors comment: 'Especially for pedophiles, vacation in a country such as Thailand apparently often provides the only opportunity for the men to realise their sexual desires' (p. 12). Men may believe that young boys, in being relatively less experienced, are unlikely to be infected with HIV.

In further work, Kleiber and Wilke (1993), conducted interviews with heterosexual and homosexual male sex tourists in a variety of destinations. A total of 661 heterosexual and 105 homosexual German men were interviewed in Kenya, Brazil, Thailand and the Philippines. The heterosexual sample contained a higher proportion of 20–40-year-olds, and homosexual inter-viewees over-represented 40–50-year-olds in comparison to the population of Germany. The sex tourists were found to be much more sexually active than at home, with an average of four partners prior to the date of the interview. Homosexual interviewees reported an average of six partners. Among heterosexual tourists visiting Kenya, Brazil and Thailand, only 45 per cent reported consistent use of condoms, and 31 per cent never used them. In the Dominican Republic, in contrast, consistent condom use was reported by 75 per cent of men, with only 10 per cent reporting never having used them. No explanation is offered of this difference, however. Among homosexual tourists, 49 per cent reported active anal sex and among these 67.5 per cent always used condoms, 15 per cent used them sometimes and 17.5 per cent never used them. For passive anal sex the picture was slightly different, with 31 per cent reporting such activity and of these 81.5 per cent consistently used condoms, while 18.5 per cent never used them.

The studies undertaken by Klieber and Wilke provide interesting information, but they focus primarily on the behaviour of tourists and the contextual factors which influence that behaviour. Little mention is made of the workers within the indigenous sex industries. More information in this respect is provided by a study of male sex workers and their male tourist clients in Bali, Indonesia, reported by Ford, Wirawan and Fajans (1993). Interviews were conducted with 20 sex workers and 19 clients, recruited through convenience sampling techniques. The interviews consisted of open-ended questions that explored knowledge of AIDS and STDs, socio-economic and demographic characteristics, sexual experience, attitudes and beliefs about condoms and other health practices. The age of the sex workers ranged from 18 to 30 years, with a median of 22.7 years. Most came from middle-class economic backgrounds, all had attended school and 20 per cent had at least some university or higher-level education. Both parental socio-economic background and educational attainment were considerably higher than for female sex workers in Bali. The client group included in this study consisted of tourists whose permanent residence was Europe (42 per cent), Australia (21 per cent), with the remainder coming from the USA, Japan and other countries. Ages ranged from 23 to 53 years, and respondents also tended to be highly educated. As a group they tended to be frequent travellers, with 80 per cent having made a previous visit to Bali, often for much longer than the length of stay for the average tourist.

Knowledge of the existence of AIDS was reported by all of the sex workers, although they often held inaccurate perceptions of the symptoms and modes of transmission of the HIV virus. Over half (55 per cent) felt that they were at risk of getting AIDS, and 60 per cent reported that in order to avoid this they had used condoms, whilst 40 per cent replied that they selected only 'clean' clients. In terms of condom use, 24 per cent of interviewees asked all clients to use condoms, a further 24 per cent asked those who 'looked suspicious' or they did not know, 35 per cent asked all foreign clients, and 18 per cent asked all foreign clients who were unknown to them. Condom use, therefore, appeared to be linked to beliefs about the most likely sources of HIV infection, i.e. foreigners and other clients who are in some way 'suspicious'.

Ford and Wirawan (1994) report a further study conducted between February 1992 and December 1993 of AIDS knowledge, sexual practices and sexual networks of several groups of female and male sex workers and clients in Bali. As one element of the study, one to two hour structured interviews were conducted with 80 male sex workers and 100 tourist clients of male sex workers. Tourist clients were recruited in resort areas and via sex workers. The male sex workers ranged in age from 15 to 36 years (mean 24 years). About half of the men had been working at least two years and a further 19 per cent had worked for more than a year. Many of the men had worked in other parts of Indonesia. All of the men reported tourist clients from outside of Indonesia and all reported clients from Australia, Europe or the United States. Many also reported having customers from Asian countries including Japan, Singapore, Taiwan, Hong Kong, Thailand and Korea. About half of the sex workers also reported Indonesian clients. The mean number of clients during the week before the interview was 2.8 (range 0–12). Both receptive and insertive anal intercourse were common, with 61 per cent of men reporting some form of anal sex during the previous week. Condom use was reported on an average of 48 per cent of occasions for receptive intercourse and 55 per cent for insertive intercourse (from the client's perspective, this indicates, as Wilke and Kleiber found, that condom use was more likely when they were being fucked than when clients fucked the sex worker). Sixty-one per cent of sex workers reported receptive oral sex but the mean incidence of condoms use was only 17 per cent. For insertive oral sex, the figures were 57 per cent and 14 per cent respectively. In other words, condoms were marginally more likely when the sex workers were sucking than when they were being sucked.

Tourist clients of sex workers ranged in age between 23 and 71 years with a mean age of 38.4 years. Twenty-six per cent were from Australia, 60 per cent from Europe, 8 per cent from the USA and the remainder from other countries. Table 3.2. reports the percentages of the sample who had visited other countries during the previous two years and had paid for sex in that place.

The tourist clients reported an average of 1.7 paid partners and 0.3 unpaid partners during the week before the interview while in Bali. Anal intercourse at least once was reported by 53 per cent of the tourists, with 75 per cent reporting condom use during receptive intercourse and 69 per cent during insertive intercourse. Oral sex at least once was more common (83 per cent), but condom use during this activity was very low (5–7 per cent).

Table 3.2 Travel histories and payment for sex among 100 male tourist clients of male sex workers in Bali

Place visited last two years	Percentage of visitors to that place	Percentage of visitors who paid for sex
Thailand	46	69
India	9	22
Other Asia	44	25
North America	28	11
South America	13	31
Australia	7	14
Europe	61	18

Only one UK clinic based research project reports evidence on the sexual activities of gay men abroad. Daniels *et al.* (1992) studied the issue of travel and sexually transmitted diseases (STDs) among patients attending the departments of HIV/Genitourinary Medicine at Charing Cross and Westminster Hospitals (London). Two hundred and fifty patients completed anonymous questionnaires and 243 were analysable. The sample consisted of 116 women (average age 27.2 years) and 127 men, of whom 62 were heterosexual (average age 30.6 years) and 65 were homosexual (average age 32.5 years). Ninety women, 53 heterosexual men and 53 homosexual men had travelled abroad during the previous six months. The study found that 51 per cent of heterosexual men and 36 per cent of homosexual men reported sexual intercourse with a local contact while abroad, compared with only 20 per cent of women. Partners abroad were divided into those that were 'casual' and those that were 'regular', and 36 per cent of heterosexual men, 26 per cent of homosexual men and 9 per cent of women reported sex with casual partners. Patients were also asked about condom use with both types of partner. Seventy five per cent (6 of 8) of women with casual partners had unprotected sex, compared with 42 per cent (8 of 19) of heterosexual men and 29 per cent (4 of 14) of homosexual men. Daniels *et al.* conclude that 'unsafe, casual encounters abroad are common' and that 'strategies for risk reduction in the form of education and safer sex advice is necessary for holiday makers planning to have sex abroad'.

Tveit, Nilsen and Nyfors (1994) studied possible 'import' routes of HIV infection to Norway by obtaining information on sexual contacts abroad and behavioural risk factors from patients attending an STD clinic. A questionnaire was administered to 599 new patients visiting a clinic in Bergen between April and June 1989 (411 men and 188 women). Respondents were grouped into four categories: sex with a prostitute during the last five years (62); homosexuals and bisexuals (22); prostitutes/intravenous drug users (21); and other heterosexuals (497). All respondents who mentioned sexual contact(s) abroad during the previous five years were questioned as to the country/countries where this activity took place, whether or not a condom had been used and if they were drunk when the contact had occurred.

In the total sample, 41 per cent of respondents reported a casual sexual partner abroad but this varied considerably across the four groups distinguished. Among those reporting sex with prostitutes (all men), 93 per cent reported a casual sexual partner, as did 67 per cent of IVDUs/prostitutes, 64 per cent of homosexuals/bisexuals and 33 per cent of 'other heterosexuals'. While the number of homosexuals/bisexuals in the sample was rather small, it is interesting to note that 50 per cent reported casual sex in one other country, 21 per cent in two, 7 per cent in three and 21 per cent in four or more

other countries during the previous five years. Homosexuals/bisexuals reported causal sex in northern European countries (50 per cent), southern
European countries (32 per cent), or the USA (9 per cent) with no other
country outside the western world mentioned. The authors note that in
northern European countries the majority of cases of infection continue to be
among gay/bisexual men. Patients reporting sex with prostitutes, in contrast,
showed a much wider spread of destinations in which they had casual partners
both paid and unpaid. Thus, casual sex was reported by 66 per cent of this
group in northern Europe (especially Denmark and Germany), 29 per cent in
Asia and 11 per cent in Africa.

Among the men who paid for sex, 66 per cent were either always or
sometimes drunk when having casual sex and only 15.5 per cent always used
a condom with a partner abroad. Amongst the male IVDUs, over 85 per cent
were always or sometimes drunk when having sex, and 21 per cent always used
a condom with a partner abroad. Corresponding figures for homosexuals/
bisexuals were 78 per cent of men reporting some level of drunkenness and
40 per cent always used a barrier protection abroad. There is some evidence,
therefore, that Norwegian homosexual men were more likely to report
consistent condom use compared with heterosexual men who paid for sex and
male IVDUs (data for 'other' male heterosexuals is not reported), nevertheless, there was still 60 per cent of the homosexual group reporting sex
abroad who did not use condoms consistently and in the main they were
visiting northern European countries where, as noted above, infections rates
are higher among gay men.

Merino *et al.* (1990), investigated sexual practices and contact with
foreigners amongst men attending a clinic for HIV testing in Colombia, South
America. Over a period of two years, 294 Colombian homosexual men
answered a questionnaire on sexual practices, travel abroad and contact with
foreign men, and consented to HIV-1 antibody testing. The aims of the study
were to identify associations between sexual practices and seropositivity and to
describe the epidemiologically relevant sexual practices amongst homosexual
men which may contribute to the pattern of the AIDS epidemic in Colombia.

The mean age of the sample was 27.8 years, and 21 per cent were found
to be HIV positive. Twenty-four per cent of subjects reported engagement in
predominantly insertive homosexual intercourse, whereas 76 per cent reported some level of receptive intercourse. Subjects reporting either predominantly receptive, or mixed receptive-insertive intercourse, were found to have
a seropositivity rate of 24 per cent, compared with 10 per cent of those who
reported predominantly insertive intercourse. Among men reporting contact
with foreign visitors to Colombia, 29.5 per cent were positive, compared with
17 per cent of those who had had no contact with visitors. This association also
appeared when men reporting predominantly receptive intercourse were
considered separately. However, those reporting contact with foreign visitors

also tended to have more sexual partners and were more likely to engage in receptive intercourse. Consequently, a number of factors enhancing risk were confounded in the analyses undertaken. Higher numbers of sexual partners (>10 within the previous year) and foreign travel were also associated with a higher incidence of HIV infection – both in the total sample and among men preferring receptive intercourse – but these relationships were not statistically significant. Unfortunately, no information was collected in this study on levels of condom use during intercourse.

Conclusions

It is difficult to reach any broad conclusions on the basis of the research studies reviewed for several reasons: the studies are very diverse with respect to methodology; they were conducted at different times, in different countries and in diverse settings; methods of sampling and sample sizes also vary (and in some studies the sampling is on a self-referral basis and sample sizes are very small), and variables included also vary from study to study. In two studies no distinction was drawn between receptive and insertive intercourse and in one no information was collected on condom use. It is also the case that most of the studies have methodological flaws which make it difficult to have confidence in the conclusions that the researchers reach from their data. Only the studies in Bali by Ford and her associates provide an ethnographic context to the work undertaken with sex workers and clients; the remaining studies are highly quantitative and provide very little insight into the social and inter-personal realities of sexual encounters between men in the context of travel. This is perhaps to be expected of clinic based interview/questionnaire studies, but it is especially disappointing that the field work undertaken by Kleiber and Wilke in four very different cultural contexts, provides no ethnographic information on the settings in which sex took place and the specific inter-personal and communication issues raised around negotiating sexual relation-ships between tourists and members of the host communities.

There are, in fact, striking disjunctures between the material reported in academic research papers and the pictures provided (literally and figuratively) by gay travel brochures, travel guides, and travel features in the gay press. In the latter we find concrete images of young and beautiful men in groups, enjoying themselves on the beach, in bars, in discos and in saunas. We find gay men and lesbians participating in significant gay cultural events that serve to reinforce a sense of solidarity, collective pride and participation in the making of gay culture and history. Such material is often set within the context of clear messages promoting safer sex practice. In the research reports, in contrast, we seemingly have *individual* men spanning a wide age range, with an average age in the mid- to late-30s. The focus in several accounts is on sex for payment, rather than consensual sex with local people or other tourists, and there are suggestions that travel may be motivated in some cases by paedophile interests. An issue which does appear across all reports is the substantial level of unprotected anal sex in the context of travel abroad (18–60 per cent), with a consistent tendency for the incidence of unprotected insertive sex to be higher (in the region of 32 per cent) than unprotected receptive intercourse (18–25 per cent). This suggests that tourists see receptive sex as riskier to themselves than insertive sex, but may also indicate a greater regard for personal protection than for the welfare of their partners.

The clinic samples are clearly not representative of a wider population in respect of condom use, since risk behaviour, or the consequences of it, are prime motivations for attending such clinics, but the data are indicative of continued risky practices among male travellers and tourists who seek sex with men. Nor are the studies conducted *in situ* representative of a wider population of gay travellers since such studies have targeted men paying for sex. Nevertheless, similar levels of unsafe practice emerge as for the clinic studies. Thus, the available evidence, despite its limitations, demonstrates a continuing and substantial level of unsafe sexual practice among non-representative samples of men having sex with men in the context of international travel. These findings support the need for sexual health and HIV prevention initiatives targeted at 'gay' men. More importantly, however, they indicate that larger scale, ethnographic studies of travel and sexual activity among more broadly representative samples of gay men are required which would locate information on sexual health risks within the social and cultural realities of gay tourism highlighted in the first half of this chapter. Such research would establish whether HIV prevention initiatives aimed at 'gay tourists', of the kind recently launched by *Gay Men Fighting AIDS*, are indeed required, and the data gathered would serve to refine the strategy, materials and messages involved in such campaigns.

References

ALCORN, K. (1995) (Ed.) *AIDS Reference Manual*, London: NAM Publications.

ALDRICH, R. (1993) *The Seduction of the Mediterranean: Writing, Art and Homosexual Fantasy*, London: Routledge.

ANDERSON, R.M. (1993) 'Epidemiological patterns of AIDS and HIV transmission in Europe', in BARON, C. and BUTLER, A. (Eds) *Report of the 1993 Conference of European Community Parliamentarians on HIV/AIDS*, London: All-Party Parliamentary Group on AIDS.

AUSTEN, R. (1983) 'Stoddard's little tricks in *South Sea Idyls*', *Journal of Homosexuality*, **15** 73–81.

BASHFORD, K. (1995) 'March of the stilettos', *Attitude*, January, 86–90.

BLEYS, R. (1993) 'Homosexual exile: The textuality of the imaginary paradise, 1800–1980', *Journal of Homosexuality*, **25**, (1/2), 165–182.

BRÖRING, G. (1995) 'International tourists: A specific target group for AIDS prevention programmes', in CLIFT, S. PAGE, S. and CLARK, N. (Eds) *Health and the International Tourist*, London: Routledge.

CARTER, S. (1994) 'Places of danger and places of safety: Travellers' social construction of risky locations in relation to HIV/AIDS,' paper presented at AIDS in Europe: The Behavioural Aspect Conference, Berlin.

CHANG-MUY, F. (1993) 'The human right of movement and asylum', in DEUTSCHE AIDS-HILFE (Ed.) *Migrants, Ethnic Minorities and AIDS*, Frankfurt/Main: Mabuse-Verlag.

CLARK, N. and CLIFT, S. (1995) 'Dimensions of holiday experiences and their health implications: findings from research with British tourists in Malta', in CLIFT, S., PAGE, S. and CLARK, N. (Eds) *Health and the International Tourist*, London: Routledge.

COHN, S.E., KLEIN, J.D., MOHR, J.E., HORST, C.M. and WEBER, D.J. (1994) 'The geography of AIDS: patterns of urban and rural migration', *Southern Medical Journal*, **87**(6), 599–606.

CONWAY, S., GILLIES, P. and SLACK, R. (1990) *The Health of Travellers*, Nottingham Department of Public Health Medicine and Epidemiology, University of Nottingham and Nottingham Health Authority.

COXON, P.M. (1992) 'Homosexual response studies: International report', unpublished report, Department of Sociology, University of Essex.

DANIELS, D.G., KELL, P., NELSON M.R. and BARTON, S.E. (1992) 'Sexual behaviour among travellers, *International Journal of STD's and AIDS*, **3**, 437–8.

FORD, K. and WIRAWAN, D.N. (1994) 'AIDS risk behaviours and sexual networks of male and female sex workers and clients in Bali, Indonesia', unpublished paper, Department of Population Planning and International Health, School of Public Health, University of Michigan.

FORD, N. and EISER, R. (1995) 'Risk and liminality: the HIV-related socio-sexual interaction of young tourists,' in CLIFT, S., PAGE, S. and CLARK, N. (Eds) *Health and the International Tourist*, London: Routledge.

FORD, K., WIRAWAN, D. and FAJANS P. (1993) 'AIDS knowledge, condom beliefs and sexual behaviour among male sex workers and male tourist clients in Bali, Indonesia', *Health Transition Review*, **3**(2), 191–204.

FORD, N., MATHIE E. and INMAN, M. (1995) 'Interaction to enhance mindfulness: positive strategies to increase tourist awareness of HIV and sexual health risks on holiday', in CLIFT, S. PAGE, S. and CLARK, N. (Eds) *Health and the International Tourist*, London: Routledge.

GARLAND, F.C., GARLAND, C.F., GORHAM, E.D., MILLER, M.R., CUNNION, S.O., BERG, S.W. and BALAZS, L.L. (1993) 'Lack of association of Human Immunodeficiency Virus seroconversion with visits to foreign ports in US Navy personnel', *Archives of International Medicine*, **153**, 2685–91.

GELDER, L.V. and BRANDT, P.R. (1992) *Are You Two ... Together? A Gay and Lesbian Guide to Europe*, London: Virago.

GILLIES, P. and SLACK, R. (1995) 'Context and culture in HIV prevention: the importance of holidays?', in CLIFT, S., Page, S. and CLARK, N. (Eds) *Health and the International Tourist*, London: Routledge.

GMFA (1994) 'Cumming Away Campaign', F*** sheet No. 11, 6.

GOULD, P. (1993) *The Slow Plague: A Geography of the AIDS Pandemic*, Oxford: Blackwell.

HAWKES, S. (1992) 'Travel and HIV/AIDS', *AIDS Care*, **4**(4), 446–49.

HAWKES, S.J. and HART, G.J. (1993) 'Travel, migration and HIV', *AIDS Care*, **5**(2), 207–14.

KING, E. (1993) *Safety in Numbers: Safer Sex and Gay Men*, London: Cassell.

KLEIBER, D. and WILKE, M. (1993) 'Sexual behaviour of German (sex-) tourists', paper presented at the IXth International Conference on AIDS, Berlin.

LEWIS, N.D. and BAILEY, J. (1993) 'HIV, international travel and tourism: global issues and Pacific perspectives', *Asia and Pacific Journal of Public Health*, **6**(3), 159–67.

LUONGO, M. and HOLCOMB, B. (1995) 'Geographical aspects of gay tourism in the USA', unpublished paper, Department of Urban Studies and Community Health, Edward J. Bloustein School of Planning and Public Policy, Rutgers, The State University of New Jersey.

MÅRDH, P-A. (1994) 'Does sexual risk taking increase in females during travelling?', paper presented at AIDS in Europe: The Behavioural Aspect Conference, Berlin.

MERINO, N., SANCHEZ, R.L., MUNOZ, A., PRADA, G., GARCIA, C.F. and POLK, F. (1990) 'HIV-1, sexual practices, and contact with foreigners in homosexual men in Colombia, South America', *Journal of Acquired Immune Deficiency Syndromes*, **3**, 330–4.

MERTENS, T.E., BURTON, A., STONEBURNER, R., SATO, R., BEER, D.L., CARAEL, M. and Belsey, E. (1994) 'Global estimates and epidemiology of HIV infections and AIDS', *AIDS*, **8** (suppl 1), S361–S372.

POIRIER, G. (1993) 'French Renaissance travel accounts: images of sin, visions of the new world', *Journal of Homosexuality*, **25**(3), 215–29.

POLLAK, M., DÜR, W., VINCINEAU, M., PERREAULT, M., PRUSA, R., FOUCHARD, J., BOCHOW, M., STALSTROM, O., HERRN, R., DAVIES, P., VALLIANATOS, G., KERRIGAN, CH., ALLEGRINI, F., SASSE, H., TIELMAN, R., PRIEUR, A., ANDREU, O.G., HENRIKSSON, B. and MASUR, J.B. (1994) 'Evaluating AIDS prevention for men having sex with men: The West European experience', *Sozial- und Praventivemedzin*, **39**, (Suppl 1), S47–S60.

SCHILLER, N.G., CRYSTAL, S. and LEWELLEN D. (1994) 'Risky business: the cultural construction of AIDS risk groups', *Social Science and Medicine*, **38**(10), 1337–46.

SEATON, V. (1994) (Ed.) *Tourism: The State of the Art*, Chichester: Wiley.

SMITH, R. (1994) 'Fag dance city,' *Gay Times*, **191**, 96–8.

STEARS, D. (1995) 'Travel health promotion: advances and alliances', in CLIFT, S., PAGE, S. AND CLARK, N. (Eds) *Health and the International Tourist*, London: Routledge.

TII (1994) 'Focus on the gay market', *Tourism Industry Intelligence*, **2**(1), 3.

TVEIT, K-S., NILSEN, A. and NYFORS, A. (1994) 'Casual sexual experience abroad in patients attending an STD clinic at high risk for HIV infection', *Genitourinary Medicine*, **70**, 12–14.

WELLINGS, K. (1994) 'General population. In assessing AIDS/HIV prevention: What do we know in Europe?', *Sozial- und Praventivmedizin*, **39** (Suppl. 1), S1–S111.

WILKE, M. and KLEIBER, D (1992) Sexual behaviour of gay German (sex) tourists in Thailand', Poster presented at VI International AIDS Conference/III STD World Congress, Amsterdam.

Chapter 4

Sexual Behaviour in Gay Men: Towards a Sociology of Risk

Graham Hart and Mary Boulton

In the early years of the AIDS epidemic, epidemiological studies succeeded in establishing the primary transmission routes of a possible AIDS-associated infectious pathogen, later identified as human immunodeficiency virus (HIV), and were able to determine the *risk behaviours* associated with the disease. With the development of the HIV antibody test a more detailed understanding of transmission was achieved, as the presence of infection could be determined in individuals, and the rate of infection could be determined in categories of people with shared characteristics (*risk groups*) and, though technically more subject to error, in whole populations. In this way the *relative risk* of transmission for each behaviour could be measured, refining even further the quantitative assessment of risk of infection.

What this meant for gay men was that unprotected receptive anal intercourse was recognized to be the primary risk factor for infection, with other behaviours (insertive anal and receptive oro-genital sex) being associated with reduced, but nevertheless, identifiable, risk. Thus, gay men were initially advised by doctors to refrain from any penetrative sexual activity entirely. Subsequently, the concept of 'safer sex' was developed by gay men to encompass sexual activities with significantly lower risk of infection, and these included the use of condoms in anal intercourse to reduce the likelihood that the virus, if present, would pass from one person to another.

This essentially epidemiological account of risk for HIV infection, while informing us of the 'mechanical' dynamics of transmission (excluding biological parameters such as infectivity, or individual susceptibility) does not address an entirely separate, but equally significant dimension of risk, notably how and why this occurs to particular individuals, in specific contexts and at certain times. That is, it cannot (and is not intended to) inform our understanding of the social determinants of risk.

The sociological understanding of risk encompasses the historical goal of much sociology – to establish the link between individuals and the broader social structure, making that link plausible through empirical and theoretical coherence. This means using a perspective that does not make the individual an isolated unit acting without reference to his/her surroundings, other people or larger environment, but one that accounts for risk precisely in terms of the person's immediate and broader social location and context. The aim here is not to deny human volition, but rather to assert that risk is influenced by, and has implications for, other people and wider social organization and institutions.

The aim of this chapter is to consider current research on sexual behaviour, particularly amongst gay and bisexual men, in order to make suggestions for designing research that can illuminate the social determinants of risk of HIV infection. This is part of a longer term enterprise, namely the development of a sociology of risk that can account for and explain risk in terms of community membership and social structural location.

Individual versus Social Explanations

The first point to note is that to date many of the studies in this area take the individual as the focus of research attention. Even though data are reported on a group basis, the primary aim has been to describe the particular features of individuals who engage in risk behaviours. These features can be demographic (age, geographic location, ethnicity), socio-economic (income, education, housing tenure), behavioural (reported sexual activity, use of alcohol/drugs), psychological (self-efficacy, depression, locus of control) and, on occasions, contextual (sex in bathhouses, by partner type, with condoms un/available) (Hart, 1989). Analysis takes the form of the selection of unprotected anal intercourse or known HIV infection as the dependent variable(s), with cross-tabulations and multivariate analysis identifying which of the selected independent variables correlate with increased likelihood of risk behaviour (e.g. young, poor, black, drug users with low self-esteem having sex with casual partners in public sex settings).

The value of these studies over the past 10 years has been in the way they have monitored the changes in risk behaviour as the epidemic has progressed. A reading of this literature indicates that the response by researchers to the HIV/AIDS epidemic in homosexual and bisexual men in the developed world has had three phases. In the first, researchers aimed to provide the basic epidemiological information that could help determine the degree of risk associated with particular activities, contexts and amongst some men rather than others. In the second phase they demonstrated that gay men were able to make changes in their sexual behaviour and that this could result in substantial reduction in the absolute and relative rates of HIV transmission and other sexually transmitted disease. In the third, most recent and still developing, phase they have alerted us to the possibility of continuing infection as a result either of new risk behaviour by men just beginning their sexual career, continuing risk behaviour amongst men who have always engaged in risk behaviour or renewed risk behaviour amongst men who have not maintained safer sex practices.

Such studies have been limited, however, in how far they have contributed to a sociological understanding of risk in relation to HIV infection. In restricting themselves to psychological or at best social psychological parameters of human action they have failed to take account of social dimensions beyond membership of a 'peer group'. In this schema socio-economic location, age and ethnicity are simply descriptive variables included with others in statistical analyses rather than what they really are – shorthand terms for complex and multi-dimensional social processes and experiences. Engaging with these in any meaningful way is a difficult and challenging enterprise, but one which can be productive in terms of extending the social understanding of risk. Here, we will examine different paradigms used to explain patterns of risk behaviour in research on sexual behaviour, particularly amongst gay and bisexual men, and consider their strengths and limitations in the broader enterprise of understanding – and intervening to change – the risk of HIV infection in Britain.

Relapse: a Psycho-social View of Risk

A feature of the large studies of gay male behaviour has been that respondents are recruited to prospective cohort studies. The men are regularly approached to provide information on their most recent behaviour, which can then be compared with their earlier accounts. By undertaking such analyses it became clear to researchers that not all men had 'maintained' safer sex. The term 'relapse' was introduced to describe the behaviour of that minority of men who had initially adopted safer sex behaviours but, at some point during follow-up, had had at least one episode of unprotected penetrative anal intercourse (Stall *et al.*, 1990). It appeared that a 'new' category of men had been uncovered – those who revert back to their 'former' sexual ways in the later stages of the epidemic.

The methodological and conceptual bases of the concept 'relapse' have been criticized in detail elsewhere (Davies, 1992; Hart *et al.*, 1992), and a lively debate continues over the appropriateness of this term (Davies, 1993; Ekstrand *et al.*, 1993; Kippax *et al.*, 1993). However, it is worth noting here in relation to risk behaviour that the term serves to encapsulate and express the individualized focus of much behavioural work in the AIDS field generally, and on gay men in particular. That is, it uses an expression in common use in medicine to describe the course of a pathology which may progress, remit or return. When applied to sexual behaviour, the effect is to locate the explanation for the 'deterioration' in behaviour firmly with processes internal to the individual. This, in turn, has given rise to the unintended but evident pathologizing of individual men as being prone to a weakening of the resolve to maintain safer sexual practices and to succumbing to the temptations of unprotected intercourse.

Relationships, Rules and Strategies: Risk Behaviour as Social Action

A more sociological view of risk behaviour casts it as social action, endowed with meaning and negotiated within a social environment. While research within this paradigm begins with the individual, it focuses on investigating the meaning of the behaviour to that individual and its origins within social relationships.

One of the most striking and consistent findings of behavioural research on gay men in both Britain and the USA is that high risk sex is more frequently reported with someone described as a 'regular' partner or lover (Fitzpatrick *et al.*, 1990; Hunt *et al.*, 1992). An important approach to investigating the reasons for this has been to look at the nature of regular and non-regular relationships which might give unprotected intercourse different meanings in the two contexts. For example, in our own study of 677 homosexually active men (McLean *et al.*, 1994) we found that about half had had unprotected intercourse during the previous year. The majority of men who had had unprotected intercourse with non-regular partners perceived their behaviour as not risky, despite not knowing their partner's HIV status. The main difference between regular and non-regular relationships was the degree of emotional involvement the respondents reported. Three quarters of the men were in love with their regular partner and two thirds were committed to the relationship continuing indefinitely. By contrast, very few men reported emotional involvement with non-regular partners. In a qualitative study of a subsample of these men currently under review, unprotected intercourse in the context of a regular relationship was described as a way of expressing the love and commitment to a shared life that the men felt. Unprotected intercourse with non-regular partners was described in very different terms.

Another example of research within this paradigm is provided by Hickson *et al.* (1992). Taking a sample of gay men in relationships with regular partners, the study describes the rules that couples make regarding sexual behaviour. These rules differentiate amongst sexual activities, partners and contexts, giving particular meanings to each and functioning as a joint strategy to maintain their mutual sexual health. Strategies were articulated and openly negotiated – perhaps unusually, as open communication regarding sexual matters may be the exception rather than the norm. Rules varied according to situation, but were generated jointly and explicitly to attain an agreement best suited to the participants. However, the important point here is that the identification of such rule making, which allows for and facilitates the form that sexual activity takes in different circumstances, could not have occurred in research which took as its epistemological unit of analysis the individual alone.

Our study of bisexual men (Boulton *et al.*, 1991, 1992) provides a third example of research that looks at risk taking as social action. Sexual risk behaviour with male and female partners was investigated in a sample of 60 behaviourally bisexual men. Patterns of risk behaviour differed according to the 'sexual context' in which the men lived. In particular, men who lived in a heterosexual context had quite consciously adopted the strategy of restricting themselves to safer sex with their male partners, in order to continue unrestricted sexual activities with their female partners, amongst whom condom use was not expected and might require 'explanation'. Perhaps the most significant feature of this study for research on risk is in its attempt to link the behaviour of individual men to broader social institutions, in this case the gay, bisexual and heterosexual communities. Patterns of values, norms and expectations within those 'communities' both give meaning to sexual behaviour and constrain the individual men's behavioural choices. They also mean that men and women linked to those communities have different likelihoods of exposure to HIV infection.

Kippax *et al.* (1992), in Australia, found that men who identified strongly with a gay identity were more likely to engage in safer sex than men on the periphery of, or not engaging in, an identifiable gay scene, who were not 'out' and whose primary public sexual identity was not gay. Again, these and other features of male same sex activity may be crucial in understanding sexual risk taking, even though it may be empirically challenging to link notions such as 'gay community involvement' to individualized risk behaviour. Nevertheless, so rarely has it been attempted – beyond unsupported rhetoric which asserts rather than investigates such relationships – that taking up the challenge could prove extremely fruitful.

Resources and Power: Material Constraints on Individual Behaviour

Approaches that focus exclusively on the individual are most often criticized by sociologists because of their implicit assumption of unrestricted volition in the populations studied. Behavioural choices, it is argued, are not freely made by individuals but are limited by the constraints of the situation and the resources available. Such an approach is perhaps best illustrated by research on sex workers which draws attention to the role of material resources, and the power relations that they give rise to, in determining the outcome of sexual encounters in terms of safe and unsafe sex.

Robinson and Davies (1991) contrasted two groups of male sex workers – 'rent boys' and 'call-men'. Rent boys tended to be young working class men who did not self-identify as gay, and sold sex on the streets and key bars of central London to willing 'punters'. They were characterized as having few personal resources in terms of accommodation, secure income and non-sex related labour market skills. Call-men, on the other hand, worked as escorts and masseurs, either from their own home or an agency. They could take clients home or travelled to client's homes or hotel rooms. The call-men were of middle-class backgrounds and self-identified as gay.

Systematic differences between these two groups were observed in relation to risk behaviour which were in turn related to differing access to material resources. Anal intercourse rarely took place between call-men and their clients, but condoms were used when this occurred. Penetrative sex was much more common amongst rentboys and condom use less frequent. Call-men had no need to find clients who would let them stay the night, and spent no more than an hour to an hour and a half with clients; rent boys were often looking for temporary accommodation which could mean a night with a punter. Price negotiation was more clearly undertaken prior to sex in the case of call men, whereas there was much more variability in pricing and negotiation amongst rent boys, and between them and their clients. The call men, as with female sex workers, made a major distinction between sex at work and in their 'private' lives, and were more likely to engage in unprotected intercourse with lovers and non-paying others in order to distinguish between activity with punters and friends. The rent boys had less scope for such distinctions and less control over the content of sexual encounters in different contexts.

Further work on differences amongst those who engage in street based work has been undertaken by Davies, Sandys and Feldman (1993). Comparisons between male sex workers in London and South Wales found that workers in London were more likely to depend entirely on their income from sex work, identify and socialize as rent-boys and make more use of health services. Street workers in South Wales reported more anal intercourse with clients, and were less likely to use condoms when they did so. They also charged clients less for sexual services. In a study of rent boys in Glasgow, McKeganey *et al.* (1990) suggested that amongst those young men who received payment *after* the sexual act, with little or no negotiation prior to the encounter, there was little control available to the sex workers to determine the content and nature of the activities undertaken.

These studies demonstrate the heterogeneity of social experience evident within apparently homogenous categories (sex work, street work), and this accords with sociological understanding of community dynamics, shared meanings and structural location. In relation to the latter, what these studies show also is the central role of material resources in constraining individual choice regarding risk behaviours. Where the sex worker is able to command significant resources, he is able to the negotiate price, content and organization of the sexual encounter and it is possible in most circumstances to avoid penetrative anal intercourse altogether or ensure condoms are used. Amongst young men without the personal economic resources (including access to a telephone, their own stable accomodation) power is more obviously in the hands of the punters, in particular where accomodation is being offered. Cold, hungry and desperate for a place to sleep, a utilitarian decision will be taken to opt for the temporary but tangible comforts of a hot meal and warm bed, even if this means having unsafe sex.

Policies, Power and Social Institutions: The Importance of Social Structure

Most empirical sociological research on sexual behaviour has been conducted within the paradigms described above. Patterns of risk behaviour have been described and explained in terms of the meanings of the activities and the constraints on behaviour that derive from the men's immediate social context. Few studies have attempted to go beyond this level of explanation.

A notable exception to this has been feminist research on sexual behaviour amongst women (Holland *et al.*, 1991, 1992). For sociological research on risk, perhaps the most significant contribution of feminist research is in the central role it gives to gendered imbalances in power in heterosexual relationships. The relative powerlessness of women derives not only from differences in material resources of individual men and women but from differences in the social position of men and women which are institutionalized in society.

Power imbalances are also evident in relationships between gay men. Davies *et al.*, (1993) of Project Sigma have analysed sexual relations between younger and older men and found that younger men were significantly more likely to be the receptive partner than older men. This is not a suggestion that being the receptive partner is evidence of social passivity, but that the systematic finding of such a difference across the age cohort indicates a patterned sexual response associated with power imbalance, and in this case it is age (which in itself can be indicative of increased social resources) rather than gender which is the basis of that imbalance.

Social structural determinants of risk behaviour and exposure to risk associated with power imbalances are evident again in paid sex work. For example, a bar-girl in Thailand whose rural family has taken out a loan from a brothel-owner, charging an exorbitant interest rate, will not be in a position to insist upon any condition of employment, including condom use, unless this is the accepted norm amongst other employers, employees and their clients. However, economic coercion is not the only factor determining the nature of paid sexual activity. Power is mediated directly through the social organization of any particular activity, and this was certainly evident in a study of prostitution in Central America.

Kane (1992) undertook a study on the social organization of prostitution in Belize, and this is a good example of a perspective that starts not with the individual prostitutes, but with the social and economic situation in which paid sexual encounters occur. Belize was formerly a British colony and until recently served as a base for British Defence Forces. There are a number of brothels providing sexual services for British military personnel, many of whom are there for no more than six months. A combination of the interests of senior military personnel, Belize government officials and brothel owners has ensured that, for the most part, condoms are used in the brothels; STD control measures are robust and, with the prevalence of HIV infection being reportedly low, little HIV transmission is likely to occur. However, alongside this highly organized and strictly policed system there is another, less well controlled situation involving what Kane calls 'quasi prostitution'. That is women, and some men, who visit bars frequented by British soldiers, in order to exchange sex for money or goods, perhaps over a period of several months. Whereas the economic element of the brothel sex is absolutely clear, in the situation of 'quasi prostitutes' this is implicit and couched in terms of a 'good time', whether for one night or longer. Here condom use is reportedly minimal, as the circumstances encourage the notion that a private personal, rather than a public, economic transaction is occurring. Yet the economic basis of the relationship is primary, if not as visible and 'open' as the direct money-based exchange of brothel prostitution.

Kane's research was part of a larger study on the planning of AIDS interventions for Belize, and she was able to see the effect of the distribution of her report in the country. The outcome was unfortunate, with the principal brothel in Belize City being designated as off-limits to military personnel, despite the suggestion that this was a primarily safe sex context. Kane suggested that this could increase the level of quasi-prostitution, and therefore unsafe sex with all its sexual health consequences. However, for our purposes the study is informative in that the primary focus was not individualized risk behaviour but the effect of powerful administrative structures (including the military and central government) on the social organization of sexual behaviour, even though this did not evidence a particularly reflexive and well thought through strategy in terms of HIV risk behaviour. In starting with this perspective, the study offered insights which would not necessarily have been obtained had Kane limited her research to sex workers' sense of self-efficacy in relation to clients' sexual demands.

Towards a Sociology of Risk

In recent years, interest in the subject of risk has grown enormously. Estimates of risk have long been a feature of modern life, but in the health field this has been driven by public health and epidemiological research, which has been concerned to measure risk behaviours or exposure linked to particular disease outcomes, resulting in calculations of risk associated with frequency of exposure to the putative pathogen over time. Although these are population based studies, and are not intended to explain an aetiology in individuals, they have been translated through health education into individualized and prescriptive 'risk reduction'. 'At risk' individuals are now recommended to adopt health-enhancing 'lifestyles' in which risk exposure is minimized. This redesignation of health as an exclusively individual responsibility, with no recognition that any other factors are associated with health and illness, has helped locate risk at the centre of public health discourse, and, in the field of sexual health it has been instrumental in generating research with an individual and psychological focus.

Increasingly, sociologically informed theory and research has criticized this paradigm, although there has long been an empirical tradition in the sociology of health and illness that privileged social structural factors as explanations for health inequalities and, by implication, risk exposure. Recently, however, the concept of risk has been explored in greater detail, and is seen as having the potential to bridge the gap between individuals, communities, and the larger social structure which contextualizes and determines risk exposure. There are now a number of examples of empirical research, some of which have been described here, which render risk as more problematic than previously considered.

There is developing, therefore, a sociology of risk that fills the intellectual gap between very different epistemological perspectives. The first is the social psychological accounts of individual risk taking in 'explanatory' models, such as the Health Belief Model and Health Locus of Control. Another is the social anthropological understanding of risk in terms of pollution and *cordons sanitaires*, which delimit boundaries as to that which is acceptable and taboo, as described by Mary Douglas (1984). Across both of these are broader perspectives on the 'post-modern' period, with writers questioning why risk has become such an important feature of modern life (Beck, 1992; Giddens, 1990). These analyses take us towards a sociology of risk, but there is a need to establish a body of empirical literature that unifies sociological interest in the arena of risk and sexual health.

Methodologically, the opportunities for a sociological perspective in empirical research results in certain suggestions as to the direction studies on risk might take. Here we have identified three broad organizing principles that offer a guide to future endeavour. The first of these is to recognize that sexual risk behaviour is constructed as social action, with the meaning of sexual activity generated within but also determining the form that behaviour takes. This was evident through research on individuals and couples who could account for their actions in terms of such meanings, where these were relatively explicit and potentially open to disclosure and articulation as recognized strategies. Not all such 'strategies' are shared – for example, the wives of men who had sex with other men were not aware that these existed – but the principle that meaning informs social action remains a methodological imperative; these women were having sex with their husbands on the basis of an entirely different set of shared meanings and understandings. Future studies of sexual risk behaviour in relation to HIV infection need to recognize the meaning invested in sexual behaviour if they are to move beyond the simple description of numbers and 'types' of partners or acts, and take the accounts that are provided as data to be employed in the identification of such meanings.

The second area of methodological importance is that concerning external constraints on individual behaviour. Earlier it was suggested that we did not wish to deny human volition, but to suggest that risk is influenced by other people and wider social organization. Freedom of action is inevitably curtailed by social and material conditions, and this was evident in relation to paid sex work. However, this also applies to other settings where material constraints are evident. For example, in a report on community development work undertaken with gay men in public housing in Newcastle it was clear that material constraints were a significant feature of the men's lives; condoms were items beyond the budgets of those receiving state benefits and no other source of income (Prout and Deverell, in press). Isolation and deprivation were routine features of these men's lives, and significantly structured their response to HIV and notions of risk and sexual behaviour. The methodological lessons from this kind of work relate to socio-economic status not simply as a *post hoc* descriptor or variable, but as a significant mediating determinant of risk exposure.

This leads us to the third level or factor to be considered in sociological studies of risk, namely the importance of social structure and organization and their influence on risk behaviour. The main examples given here were of gendered inequalities in power and the social organization of sex work, although other aspects of structural location are worth investigating. There is increasing interest in the effects of homophobic social policy on the lives of gay men and lesbians, particularly in relation to privileged policy fields such as the family and reproductive rights, which sees homophobic structures of state policy as comparable to the structural racism, which, it is argued, is a feature of the organization of the modern state. Certainly, critical accounts of the restrictions on sex education in schools, the tardy and very limited state provision of health education for gay men, the clawing back of monies for HIV and AIDS services because there has been 'no heterosexual epidemic' and the legal restrictions placed on gay male sexuality do suggest the value of a re-consideration of homophobia as more than simply a feature of individual personality, whether as pathology or attitude (King, 1993). It may be challenging methodologically to suggest this as an area of research, connecting with lived experience and risk as reported by respondents, but it is certainly not an area of study beyond empirical scrutiny.

Conclusions

In this chapter we have suggested that there is much greater potential for research that employs a specifically sociological perspective to shed further light on sexual risk behaviour. Our concern has been primarily with research on gay men, but this approach has proven useful in studies of other populations. Early in the epidemic it was necessary to undertake descriptive work very quickly as the basic parameters of gay male sexual behaviour were simply unknown. However, there is now a need for progression beyond the individual reports of sexual activity, to an improved appreciation of the social at the heart of the sexual. By understanding that sexual acts involving two or more people are examples of social action one can then study the nature of any risk or hazard in terms of these primarily social relations. The links between people, the context in which activity occurs, and the social relations that further connect those involved to communities of interest within broader social structures are a starting point rather than an after-thought for the sociologist studying risk. With increasing interest in developing targeted interventions for gay men, which depend on community membership and shared structural location, such work will take on ever increasing significance as the epidemic matures.

References

BECK, U. (1992) *Risk Society: Towards a New Modernity,* London: Sage.
BOULTON, M., SCHRAMM-EVANS, Z., FITZPATRICK, R. and HART, G. (1991) 'Bisexual men: women, safer sex and HIV transmission', in AGGLETON, P., HART, G. and DAVIES, P. (Eds) *AIDS: Responses, Interventions and Care,* London: Falmer Press.
BOULTON, M., HART, G. and FITZPATRICK, R. (1992) 'The sexual behaviour of bisexual men in relation to HIV transmission', *AIDS Care,* 4, 165–72.

DAVIES, P. (1992) 'On relapse: recividism or rational response?', in AGGLETON, P., DAVIES, P. and HART, G. (Eds) *AIDS: Rights, Risk and Reason*, London: Falmer Press.

DAVIES, P.M. (1993) 'Safer sex maintenance among gay men: are we moving in the right direction?' *AIDS*, **7**, 279–80.

DAVIES, P.M., SANDYS, S. and FELDMAN, R. (1993) 'Patterns of male sex-work in areas of high and low HIV seroprevalence in the UK', abstract PO-DO9-3657, *IXth International Conference on AIDS/IVth STD World Congress*, Berlin, June 1993.

DAVIES, P.M., HICKSON, F.C.I., WEATHERBURN, P. and HUNT, A.J. (1993) *Sex, Gay Men and AIDS*, London: Falmer Press.

DOUGLAS, M. (1984) *Purity and Danger: An Analysis of the Concepts of Pollution and Taboo*, London: Ark.

EKSTRAND, M., STALL, R., KEGELES, S., HAYS, R., DE MAY, M. and COATES, T. (1993) 'Safer sex among gay men: what is the ultimate goal?', *AIDS*, **7**, 281–2.

GIDDENS, A. (1990) *The Consequences of Modernity*, Cambridge: Polity.

HART, G. (1989) 'AIDS, homosexual men and behavioural change', in MARTIN, C.J. and McQUEEN, D.V. (Eds) *Readings for a New Public Health*, Edinburgh: Edinburgh University Press.

HART, G., BOULTON, M., FITZPATRICK, R., McLEAN, J. and DAWSON, J. (1992) 'Relapse to unsafe sexual behaviour amongst gay men: A critique of recent behavioural HIV/AIDS research', *Sociology of Health and Illness*, **14**, 216–32.

HART, G.J., DAWSON, J., FITZPATRICK, R.M., BOULTON, M., McLEAN, J., BROOKES, M. and PARRY, J.V. (1993) 'Risk behaviour, anti-HIV and anti-HBc prevalence in clinic and non-clinic samples of gay men in England, 1991–2,' *AIDS*, **7**, 863–869.

HICKSON, F., DAVIES, P. HUNT, A.J., WEATHERBURN, P., MCMANUS, T.J. and COXON, A.P.M. (1992) 'Maintenance of open gay relationships: some strategies for protection against HIV', *AIDS Care*, **4**, 409–419.

HOLLAND, J., RAMAZANOGLU, C., SCOTT, S., SHARPE S. and THOMPSON, R. (1991) 'Between embarrassment and trust: young women and the diversity of condom use', in AGGLETON, P., HART, G. and DAVIES, P. (Eds) *AIDS: Responses, Interventions and Care*, London: Falmer Press.

HOLLAND, J., RAMAZANOGLU, C., SCOTT, S., SHARPE, S. and THOMPSON, R. (1992) 'Pressure, resistance, empowerment: young women and the negotiation of safer sex', in 'Aggleton, P., Davies, P. and HART, G. (Eds) *AIDS: Rights, Risk and Reason*, London: Falmer Press.

HUNT, A.J., DAVIES, P.M., McMANUS, T.J., WEATHERBURN, P., HICKSON, F.C.I., CHRISOFINIS, G., COXON, A.P.M. and SUTHERLAND, S. (1992) *British Medical Journal*, **305**, 561–2.

KANE, S.C. (1992) 'Prostitution and the military: Planning AIDS intervention in Belize', *Social Science and Medicine*, **36**, 965–79.

KING, E. (1993) *Safety in Numbers*, London: Cassell.

KIPPAX, S., CRAWFORD, J., CONNELL, B., DOWSETT, G., WATSON, L., RODDEN, P., BAXTER, D. and BERG, R. (1992) 'The importance of gay community in the prevention of HIV transmission: A study of Australian men who have sex with men', in AGGLETON, P., DAVIES, P. and HART, G. (Eds) *AIDS: Rights, Risk and Reason*, London: Falmer Press.

KIPPAX, S., CRAWFORD, J., DAVIS, M., RODDEN, P. and DOWSETT, G. (1993) 'Sustaining safe sex: a longitudinal study of a sample of homosexual men', *AIDS*, **7**, 257–63.

McKEGANEY, N.P., BARNARD, M.A. and BLOOR, M.J. (1990) 'A comparison of HIV-related risk behaviour and risk reduction between female street-working prostitutes and male rent boys in Glasgow', *Sociology of Health and Illness*, **12**, 274–92.

McLean, J., Boulton, M., Brookes, M., Lakhani, D., Fitzpatrick, R., Dawson, J., McKechnie, R. and Hart, G. (1994) 'Regular partners and risky behaviour: why do gay men have unprotected intercourse?', *AIDS Care*, **6**.

Prout, A. and Deverell, K. (1995) *MESMAC: Working with Diversity – Building Communities*, London: HEA/Longman.

Robinson, T. and Davies, P. (1991) 'London's homosexual male prostitutes: power, peer groups and HIV', in Aggleton, P., Hart, G. and Davies, P. (Eds) *AIDS: Responses, Interventions and Care*, London: Falmer Press.

Stall, R., Ekstrand, M., Pollack, L., McKusick, L. and Coates, T.J. (1990) 'Relapse from safer sex: the next challenge for AIDS prevention efforts', *Journal of Acquired Immune Deficiency Syndromes*, **3** 1181–7.

Chapter 5

Framing Difference:
Sexuality, AIDS and Organization

David Goss and Derek Adam-Smith

The issue of AIDS cannot be separated from persisting relations of power and influence that pervade societies and organizations. Although involving inequalities of race, disability and class, the issue that has emerged most strongly in the HIV/AIDS debate in the UK is that of sex and sexuality. However, in most organizational responses to the epidemic this matter has been largely silent, either because sex and sexuality are defined as taboo subjects within the workplace and their discussion effectively 'suppressed', or because their very existence within this sphere of supposedly rational behaviour is denied. Many recent developments in critical organization theory, however, have undermined the sustainability of such a desexualized stance. Hearn and Parkin (1987), for instance, stress the importance of 'organization sexuality', by which they mean a 'sexual structuring' whereby organizations are continually divided by sex and sexualities, one characteristic of which is the dominance of male constructions of heterosexuality over other forms of sexuality.[1]

> The dominant concrete form that heterosexuality takes in this society is an hierarchical one. Thus a major, and perhaps central, feature of the sexual 'normality' of organizations is a powerful heterosexual bias: a form of 'compulsory heterosexuality' ... the domination and oppression of homosexuality, lesbianism and other sexualities perceived as 'other'.
>
> (Hearn and Parkin, 1987: 94)

This chapter sets out to explore the ways in which HIV/AIDS is framed as an organizational issue and how these framings intersect with notions of organization sexuality. The data presented is taken from a larger set of interviews with employees and managers in a variety of organizations. As the

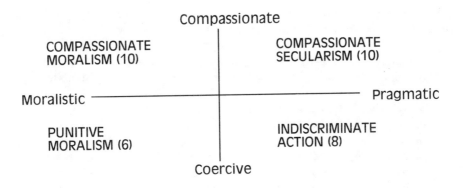

Compassionate

COMPASSIONATE
MORALISM (10)

COMPASSIONATE
SECULARISM (10)

Moralistic ———————————————————— Pragmatic

PUNITIVE
MORALISM (6)

INDISCRIMINATE
ACTION (8)

Coercive

N = 34

Figure 5.1 Herek and Glunt's typology of attitudes to AIDS

analysis of this data is still at an early stage, the present cases have been selected because they make explicit reference to the AIDS/sexual-identity/organization nexus.[2]

For the purposes of exposition we have organized our data via a 'conventional' typology of attitudes to AIDS developed by Herek and Glunt (1991),[3] although this will be subject to a rereading using concepts from Goffman's *Frame Analysis* (Goffman, 1975) in the concluding section of the chapter. It will be apparent from the following accounts that there are issues of difficulty concerning the drawing of boundaries between the typology quadrants; this is picked up in detail in the concluding discussion. The distribution of respondents between these categories is given in Figure 5.1.[4] The criteria we have used to allocate cases to categories are outlined at the beginning of each section.

Compassionate Secularism

In ideal-typical terms Compassionate Secularism is represented by beliefs that embody a commitment not to discriminate unfairly against people affected by HIV/AIDS; recognize the importance of heterosexism as an additional basis for discrimination that may be attached to AIDS; and demonstrate a commitment to gaining greater acceptance (ideally parity) of non-heterosexual identities and the lengthening of the equal opportunities agenda. A principal concern of those falling into this category was an acute awareness of the potential for prejudice resulting from misconceived links between AIDS and homosexuality. Thus, when speaking of the issues to which

AIDS could give rise in the workplace, most drew attention to the pervasiveness of homophobia. For example:

> I remember at a board meeting in my previous company a manager was almost passed over because of being gay, not because of his ability but because the way the guy wanted to live his life. But because somebody said he was gay they thought, 'Hang on fellows, what are we talking about?' The argument that ensued was quite interesting because then they started looking at other guys' behaviours, far more damming because the gay guy was very discreet, kept his private life very private and performed his job and was well respected and a good manager. Another colleague who was 'one of the boys', was in fact often an acute embarrassment because of his drinking and womanizing. But he was 'okay' and this was from board level guys. So you've got a lot of prejudice and stereotyping.
>
> (Personnel Manager, Hotel)

> We did do an exercise once about prejudice and how we could perceive people to be. You get the young-looking hairdresser and we did a group and they said he must be gay because he is a hairdresser and he is young and that's how we have perceived that person to be and yet we can be so wrong so many times and I think it's a shame.
>
> (Personnel Manager, Retail/Distribution)

> I think it's sexuality that is the problem for people and I don't think people know it. It's mixed into a lot of fear and misunderstanding about HIV and I think in terms of employing somebody with HIV, I still think most people are at the point where HIV comes along with a panic and you don't know how to control it. So I think certainly its an issue around sexual orientation, I think people have their personal prejudices around that and how they manage that.
>
> (Social Worker)

Given this awareness of heterosexual bias as a factor influencing reactions to AIDS, respondents frequently pointed to the need for education about associated sexual attitudes and values, thus:

> The THT 'Positive Management' pack was very well done. I particularly liked the non-detrimental scenario that they were putting out, very real dealing with everyday people. Characters that they were using, ordinary-looking people, everyday kinds of people saying things clearly, it kind of brought it home. I showed it to other people, it's almost like you were confronted with it and suddenly it raised an

awful lot of questions like, 'I would never have believed that guy was gay?'; 'What's he supposed to have? Three heads?', this kind of thing. It's getting rid of the stereotypes.

(Personnel Manager, Hotel)

Our experience of talking about issues of HIV and AIDS means you are talking about love and sex and all of those things which people don't tend to talk about at work. Quite a lot of barriers were broken down when we started having those conversations and I think it created a good feeling and brought us closer to each other as a result, but that was nearly a year ago. Maybe we need to do something to get that closeness back.

(Distribution Manager)

The course was held in London, that was actually presented by a chap who was gay and his partner who in fact was HIV positive, which they did not divulge until near the end, that really went in to more how people feel. That was very useful ... They were very good and effective.

(Personnel Manager, Charity)

However, despite a certain consistency, this category was by no means completely homogeneous, tending to divide between those who favoured a 'low key' and informal resolution of the AIDS-sexuality dilemma, and those who advocated open confrontation and formalization. The former response was summed up by a senior personnel manager who began by pointing to the complexities surrounding homosexual identities in heterosexually structured organizations:

I think that the most important thing is that people have got to feel okay. There are members of the gay community who are very comfortable with their sexuality and don't give a damn. There is another group which are comfortable but are not so open and there are some who are very scared and they are often fearful of what would happen if it became common knowledge that they were gay and it acts like an extra burden to carry. They assume people automatically think if they are gay then they assume they are HIV.

(Personnel Manager, Hotel)

For this respondent, the important aspect of dealing with AIDS and sexuality in the workplace was to establish a culture of trust in which all organization members would be treated as individuals and assessed on their job performance rather than on the basis of their social 'status'. This led to a scepticism towards the effectiveness of rule-making and formal policy:

> I am concerned about making any policy illness-related as in the majority of cases in our company primarily one group of people, which is the gay people, will be affected. Any legislation which focuses on one particular social group I have a problem with. It refocuses the mind on the wrong points.
>
> (Personnel Manager, Hotel)

Here sexuality was considered a matter of private identity that should properly be separate from work *role* (although not necessarily completely subsumed by a workplace *identity*). Thus, where an identity-role conflict occurred this could be dealt with on a case-by-case basis within a framework of tolerance. As this respondent explained:

> One experience I have had that was memorable, it surprised every-body ... The initial reaction was shock, horror and the disbelief that Nigel was gay. Then some embarrassment, then some guilt, like 'Why he didn't tell us?' then it goes back to shock again, because then you realise that he has got HIV and potentially that he could be dead in a certain length of time. Then there is a tremendous feeling of 'What can we do?' When the guy did die the reaction from the staff was considerable.
>
> (Personnel Manager, Hotel)

In this case, it seems, Compassion is personal and individual, and Secularism implies expurgation of sexuality from *formal* organization discourse, a stance which parallels the notion of 'hidden conflict' (Kolb and Putnam, 1992:19) whereby some issues are dealt with informally and privately and resolved by 'avoidance, accommodation, tolerance or behind-the-scenes coalition build-ing' rather than confrontation . However, whilst such a strategy could be justified on the grounds that, given existing disparities in sex-power, it is better to 'bend with the wind' than to 'snap in the breeze', it could also be objected to in some quarters (as we will see below) because it appears to acquiesce in the dominance of heterosexism (see also Cockburn, 1991).

Indeed, for another respondent, this strategy of informal accommodation was less attractive than frontal challenge to established heterosexism. AIDS, in fact, was seen as a weapon in the attempt to gain organizational acceptance of homosexual identity:

> The equal opps. policy is on the grounds of race, gender, physical ability, religion, leaves out sexual orientation and HIV status which is a terrible error, terrible omission, there's massive resistance to AIDS

... I think its a good way to get sexual orientation considered actually. I know a lot of places wouldn't normally consider that in their equal opps scheme but have as a result of having to consider HIV status ... the drawbacks are that it emphasizes feelings like the gay plague type of thing, but that's not a drawback in the long term. As long as sexual orientation gets in there, I'm not really bothered about how as long as it does. As long as its in there they can't damn you for it.

(Social Worker)

This stance placed a greater emphasis on formal recognition (including sanctions against those who proved maliciously recalcitrant) of homo-sexualities, and emphasized a commitment that this issue should be faced openly and collectively, as a social rather than a purely personal matter. This was encapsulated in the written policy of one organization where this approach was espoused:

There exists within society a negative and condemnatory response to the infection. This may be explained by society's homophobia and the early known transmission of the infection, in the west, amongst the male, homosexual community and injecting drug users ... carrying the infection remains a potentially stigmatizing and alienating experi-ence ... This policy must be read and implemented in the context of the Equal Opportunities Policy, which is applicable to staff who are HIV+ or who have AIDS. These staff are potentially subject to prejudice and disadvantage and, therefore, Equal Opportunities Policy applies to them. In assessing the needs of, and working with, people who are HIV+ or who have AIDS, the context of the person's race, culture, religious and spiritual belief and sexual orientation must be taken into account. To promote positive images of, and for, people with HIV and with AIDS and to diminish the effects of stigmatization associated with infection.

(Charity)

Indiscriminate Action

Indiscriminate Action, like Compassionate Secularism, retains a focus that is pragmatic rather than moralistic but combines this with an acceptance of coercive measures against people with HIV/AIDS. Thus, it involves an ambivalence towards AIDS with particular views informed by specific circum-stances and situations; a pragmatic 'common sense' view that homosexuality is a credible associate of HIV infection and, as such, those claiming (or suspected of having) such an identity can be legitimately regarded as targets of suspicion and perceived risk; and a preparedness to accept discriminatory measures, either against those with the virus or who could be suspected of carrying it, if there is felt to be any chance of risk to the 'healthy' population; where no such risk was apparent, a strategy of 'live and let live/die' could be adopted.

The concept of Indiscriminate Action reflects an ostensibly amoral stance guided by concerns of prudent self/other protection in the face of an uncertain hazard (Smithurst, 1990). In one case, for instance, the issue of sexual transmission was presented as a *universal* threat (rather than a matter of moral distaste), which justified HIV testing on a grand scale and workplace surveillance of sexual behaviour:

> I think something ought to be done worldwide as regards the testing of AIDS, it's a very serious thing. I think everyone should be tested, it's a frightening thing, ... [If I thought someone was HIV+] I would be wary of the fact, and keep an eye on his/her behaviour, it's like if he or she started sleeping around, you know.
>
> (Nightclub Manager)

In other cases, though, the links between AIDS, risk and sexuality were configured in terms which implicated homosexuality as an object of concern if not explicit moral condemnation. For example:

> I don't see anything against homosexuals or anything like that, but I think we ought to know, we need to be more careful about it. But they are not the only ones who carry AIDS, I mean there is a hell of a lot of other groups who carry AIDS.
>
> (Metal Worker)

This association of AIDS and homosexuality, however, did have a bearing on the sorts of 'action' that were considered appropriate for workplace settings. A benign form, for instance, involved a management decision deliberately to exclude AIDS from equal opportunities policy agendas in order to forestall raising questions of sexual orientation, this suppression of homosexual identity being justified pragmatically because of its perceived threat to other 'mainstream' policies. Thus:

> We haven't really addressed the area of equal opps relating to sexuality and AIDS. It's not something we want to raise, not because we don't want to, but we don't want to be diverted from a number of other things which we are still having to argue issues about. I mean we shouldn't have to argue women's issues in 1993. If we got diverted and we know there's going to be a lot of objections, it's not going to help

the equal opps policy, so we haven't addressed sexual health issues in the equal opps policy so far.

(Public Sector Manager)

Similar, but less clearly articulated, negative associations between homosexual identity and HIV-infection were also made by employees in health-care organizations. Here, too, the issue was one of individual tolerance outweighed by perceived disruption to organizational operations:

If members of the public found out that somebody here was HIV positive or that we were seeing AIDS patients, our practice would lose patients, I know it would. There is still a stigma attached to it. It's still the gay plague.

(Dental Assistant)

If they are a student, part of their training is how to give injections, and they go to do a bit of practice and there is a mishap, you have an injury, and there is your problem. I think the answer is that, I suppose there is no reason why they could not do the academic part of the course, but I don't know about the practical ...

We have a [gay] lad at the moment and he is lovely and the way he talks to families, he *actually* gets on quite well now. I mean *as people* they have been very nice.

(Nurse) (emphasis added, see below)

Note in the last quotation the unstated identification of the gay man as 'other than a normal person'. The question of whether this 'otherness' includes propensity to be HIV seropositive thus remains open and, as such, creates at least the potential for action to be discriminatory.

Indeed, other responses involved the open approval of surveillance and 'investigation' applied to employees known to be, or suspected of being, gay (although as one respondent noted, it was 'nothing personal'). For example:

I mean you'd want to go into their personal lives to find out if he is a homo or if this particular person does sleep around without the proper precautions.

(Metal Worker [2])

Maybe on the gay side, asking them maybe to have a urine test to make sure they haven't contracted during the time.

(Hotel Manager)

Responses in this category were not without their own tensions which, in the absence of a strong moral dimension, mostly hinged around issues of practicality. In particular, there was a 'resigned tolerance' whereby action against those perceived as likely 'carriers' of HIV was rejected on grounds of feasibility rather than principle. For instance:

> I don't think you would ever get a straight answer, certainly if you asked someone if they were a drug user. So I don't think you would ever get a straight answer if you ask somebody what their sexual persuasions are.
>
> (Hotel Manager)

> I don't know, how do you go about asking that sort of thing anyway? I don't think it is ever going to be one of those things you're going to be able to solve.
>
> (Metal Worker)

There is clearly a problem in regarding the boundaries of this group too rigidly. It was apparent that in some cases, and despite claims of amorality, there was a strong sense of disapproval towards homosexuality, evidenced by one respondent thus:

> I personally haven't, this is my personal opinion, I haven't got any time for homosexuals, they leave me alone, I'll leave them alone. And er, no they just should be treated like the rest of us. No favouritism and no discrimination.
>
> (Metal Worker [2])

It is quite possible, therefore, that this category may capture what respondents perceive to be 'respectable' answers, thereby masking views more appropriately classified as either Compassionate Moralism or Punitive Moralism.

Compassionate Moralism

Moving to the 'moral' side of the typology, Compassionate Moralism can be defined as a commitment not to discriminate unfairly against people affected by HIV/AIDS; a belief that AIDS is largely the result of 'unnatural' or irresponsible behaviour, and that those affected are, thus, not wholly without blame for their condition; the view that whilst those with AIDS/HIV should not be the subject of repressive control, neither should the behaviour be responsible for their predicament be encouraged or openly condoned; in short, they should be viewed as deserving of pity and sympathy but not unconditionally supported.

A common theme among respondents in this category was a concern to establish a sense of difference between themselves and, as one quaintly put it, those of 'a homosexual persuasion'. For instance:

> Now most people who are in a normal, god-fearing working life, like you and I, I assume, we don't really come into heavy contact with people like that, do we? Homosexuals are very clandestine because of the nature of their relationships . . . they don't live a normal life, as we know.
>
> (Metal Worker [3])

Indeed, it was the ability to maintain this difference that provided the discursive space for expressions of tolerance and sympathy. Consider the following:

> I used to like Queen [the rock group] and I thought 'Oh God! No, not him', because I think he [Freddy Mercury] was a real . . ., you know, and then it put me off of his music. So it could put me off a person, that's what I am saying, I really used to like him, and then I thought, 'Oh goodness no, what a waste of a life', or whatever, but then again, how do you know how he caught it?
>
> (Print Worker)

> It is general knowledge that homosexuals obviously transmit it [HIV] through their varied, colourful sex life . . . Not that I'm homosexual! . . . But most of it is people who are a bit frightened of them because they don't really understand them. Now, what they are doing is not what was written in the good book, so therefore it must be wrong . . . as long as they don't interfere with your life or in any way try to persuade you to their way of thinking then they should have the same rights as us, shouldn't they.
>
> (Metal Worker [3])

> I mean it was one of those things that I'd sort of put two and two together anyway just from observing him. I just had this gut feeling. You just sort of pick up vibes don't you, and I had thought he was perhaps homosexual anyway, er, he was always very pleasant, I just had that feeling.
>
> (Clerical Worker, Factory)

The last quotation picks up another theme in the maintenance of difference, namely its achievement – somewhat paradoxically – through exaggerated expressions of surprise about how normal individual homosexuals were 'really' (often along the lines of 'some of my best friends are gay'). As others illustrate:

> In Devon where I worked we had a gay bar man, he wasn't overtly gay
> he was in the closet and you know I got on fine with him, there were
> no problems.
>
> (Barman, Nightclub)

> I went on a tour of Europe and one of the guys was gay, he didn't tell
> any of us, because he thought especially the guys, might think
> differently of him; and all the girls knew, I don't know his manner, just
> his way, I mean it didn't bother us.
>
> (Barman [2], Nightclub)

> We have a gay at the moment in the coffee house and he's been there
> a long time about 18 years with the company.
>
> (Hotel Receptionist)

The quotations cited above can be seen as attempts to manage what were
perceived to be the 'spoilt' or 'discreditable' identities of others (Goffman,
1963). However, although it has often been pointed out that defining others
as 'deviant' or 'abnormal' can serve to reconfirm our own normality, the
respondents here were not working with such a simple binary divide; rather,
the normal/abnormal distinction appeared as a duality, a tension, between a
'virtual' and an 'actual' identity. It involved the assumption that a homosexual
identity was essentially 'discredited' (doubly so given its association with AIDS)
but that opportunities could be provided for such individuals to 'prove' by
their actions that *they* were not wholly so. In effect to allow them the space for
a status transformation from discredited to discredit*able* (i.e. with the potential
to be discredited), a tacit understanding to ignore – but not repudiate – the
stigmatized identity, provided other expressions of 'normality' were maintained, such a 'transformation' being facilitated by the implicit and explicit
'rules' that maintain organization sexualities (Mills and Murgatroyd, 1991).
Thus, the 'acid test' for 'discreditability' was the extent to which these
unspoken rules were obeyed. This was highlighted in the account of one
respondent who recalled a situation when the bounds of such propriety had
been overstepped:

> The only one we had here, we had a transvestite here, he was a nice
> looking chap but he liked to dress in the female dress, the only trouble
> was that he was using the women's toilet so we had to sack him.
>
> (Metal Worker [3])

> If someone came in there, if somebody came in and talking like a
> madam and with a really high voice then they might pull jokes about
> him, that type of thing I mean.
>
> (Print Worker)

It seemed, then, that the precondition for the 'toleration of difference' was an individual deference towards heterosexual 'normality' on the part of the 'other' and a suppression of deliberate expressions of homosexuality.

Punitive Moralism

The final category, Punitive Moralism, rests upon the following assumptions: AIDS is a disease resulting from fundamentally corrupt and perverse sexual behaviours; those who have the virus, and are thus implicated in such behaviour, are both a medical and a moral threat to others and should, therefore, be excluded from normal social relations, including employment; and steps to identify and discriminate against such people both at the pre- and post-employment stage are defensible and desirable.

The general tenor of responses in this category reflected a more rigid view of the discredited homosexual identity as incapable of even partial 'redemption'. This is captured by the following quotations:

> If I knew there was a homosexual here, then I would possibly, certainly protest slightly ... I would turn around and I definitely wouldn't work with the person. It might sound nasty. I don't know whether I could accept it. It's like I suppose taking your child into a house where you know someone has HIV ... with your own kid it's the last thing you'd want.
>
> (Chef, Public Sector)

> They wouldn't work here. They would be fired straight away ... there would just be an atmosphere in there all the time ... I would keep away.
>
> (Nightclub Manager)

However, in addition to an antipathy towards homosexuality these respondents also tended to exhibit low levels of understanding of HIV and, to a greater extent than other respondents, felt themselves personally to be at risk from the virus. For example:

> How can it be transmitted? Can it be transmitted on money, you know things like that, maybe it can be transmitted through food, maybe it can be transmitted through something else ...
>
> (Chef, Public Sector)

> I wouldn't like anybody behind the bar to be employed who is HIV positive, if cuts happen, constant contact with liquids that are drunk by customers, coming into contact with customers ... I wouldn't

> expect them to be handling the glassware, as far as I am concerned ...
> [Testing] wouldn't be a bad idea, I personally wouldn't give objec-
> tions if someone tested me ... Yes I would think that would be a pretty
> good thing actually. Yes, that would be good.'
>
> (Bar Manager)

> I mean even in my kind of job you are always cutting yourself on the
> metal. When you cut yourself you leave blood on the metal and the
> next person picks it up and it's, there's got to be some way to stop it
> spreading, unless I'm ignorant of that part but I think blood is one of
> the main factors.
>
> (Metal Worker [4])

An alternative response to framing these issues in terms of risk was to locate
them in relation to guilt and innocence. Thus, distinctions were made
between those who were infected with HIV 'accidentally' and those who had
contracted the virus as a result of 'unacceptable' and 'irresponsible' activity.
Thus:

> I've got a lot of sympathy for those who are heterosexual, but I haven't
> got much sympathy for homosexuals because they know what they are
> getting involved with ... I wouldn't want them touching me, well it's
> silly to say that, I would feel sorry for them depending totally on the
> circumstances ... If he was known to be very promiscuous, I wouldn't
> feel too sorry for him as he brought it on himself.
>
> (Nightclub Waitress)

> You've got more chance of getting HIV if you are homosexual than
> heterosexual. I wouldn't like to be expert on homosexuality or like
> that ... But I think gays are a high risk and they should at least check
> it out ... I'm a clean person so I know I'm okay.
>
> (Nightclub Bouncer)

Frame Analysis

A number of qualifications are now in order, however, since our typological
usage has departed significantly from that intended by the original designers
of this framework. For Herek and Glunt, this typology was a representation of
attitudes captured through specifically designed and validated measurement
scales. Our use has been more casual in that it has involved the allocation of
pieces of speech extracted from interviews to categories on the basis of an
apparent face-congruity.

We do not, in fact, consider the categorized words from our respondents as evidence of coherent attitude formations as understood by psychologists. Rather, we have found it more useful to approach these expressions through concepts developed from Goffman's frame analysis (as we have argued elsewhere, there is a strong affinity between this approach and current developments in (postmodernist) organization theory, (Burns, 1992; Goss, 1995).

Frame analysis is about how actors shape and compartmentalize the meanings of 'strips of action' which constitute the 'experience of social life', it is about how definitions of situation are built up: in short, the 'organization of experience' (Goffman, 1975). As will be explored in more detail below, the categories of the typology we present are to be understood as particular framings of AIDS/organization/sexuality discourse that, while exhibiting a certain mutual consistency, are not necessarily firmly 'fixed'. Rather they are capable of transformation and reinterpretation in a variety of ways and for various purposes depending on the situation and interests of their 'author'.

Although a precise definition of a frame is difficult to pin down in Goffman's account, Burns (1992) suggests that the simplest way to understand it is to equate it with the notion of 'mental set':

> an anticipatory response of an individual which is directed towards interpreting and assessing the situation so as to guide his own actions. To regard perception as the active probing and testing-out of the environment is axiomatic for both 'frame' and 'mental set'. Generalised schemata and prototypes composed out of previous experience are summoned as first approximations, *then refined or amended as more information is added.*
>
> (Burns, 1992: 251 with emphasis added)

By drawing attention to this 'layered' or 'laminated' quality of socially constructed meanings, frame analysis provides a useful conceptual vocabulary for the exploration of discursive activity and its effects. The principal components of this vocabulary being primary and secondary frameworks, keyings and fabrications.

Primary frameworks, according to Goffman, are schemata of interpretation, the application of which is seen by those who apply them as not depending on, or harking back to, some prior or 'original' interpretation' (Goffman, 1975: 21). Or, as Burns puts it, provide the 'organizing principle by which the world of everyday reality ... is sustained by intersubjective understanding' (1992: 251). In this respect, primary frameworks can be regarded as the 'master frame' for subsequent organizings. Primary frames, however, seldom operate in a 'pure' form or as a homogeneous organizing structure. Rather, to cope with the complexity and unpredictability of social experience, they are subject to transformation and reworking through the 'layering' of secondary frameworks. Thus:

> When the idea of framing is expanded so as to include rekeyings as well as keyings we end up with a picture of successive transformations (keyings) laid on top of each other, with the original model, which is locked into one or other primary framework, at the base. The whole construction bears a close resemblance to Ryle's 'pyramid' of increasingly sophisticated actions with each higher layer made feasible only because of all the layers of cognitive experience which have preceded it ... it is the 'outermost layer' that ties the whole activity to the 'real world.'
>
> (Burns, 1992: 257)

The utility of this approach is that it allows us to look at speech not as the expression of coherent and self-contained attitudes, but rather as a developing and inherently dynamic attempt to locate a particular issue within, and in relation to, a wider/pre-existing set of meanings of discourses. This, then, enables the conception of the boundaries between the different categories within our typology as permeable and overlapping; indeed, each one can be seen as potentially 'built' upon any other, thereby allowing a rereading of the typology as a 'stack' or laminate (such that any given position can be shifted by moving through successive layers), rather than a fixed two-dimensional matrix with mutually exclusive categories. This can be illustrated by a brief consideration of two aspects of frame analysis: 'keyings' and 'fabrications' which we will use, somewhat speculatively, to extend the scope of the typology.

The process of frame transposition, which Goffman refers to as 'keying' (based on the musical metaphor of transposing keys), involves the following elements:

> a) A systematic transformation is involved across materials already meaningful in accordance with a schema of interpretation, and without which the keying would be meaningless.
> b) Participants in the activity are meant to know and to openly acknowledge that a systematic alteration is involved, one that will radically reconstitute what for them is going on ... A keying ... performs a crucial role in determining what it is we think is really going on.
>
> (Goffman, 1975: 45)

For the purposes of illustration, four keyings and four fabrications will be discussed: (1) from compassionate secularism to indiscriminate action; (2)

from indiscriminate action to compassionate secularism; (3) from compassionate moralism to punative moralism; and (4) from punitive moralism to compassionate moralism. Each frame shift is dealt with below, first for keyings and then for fabrications.

Keyings

The keying from Compassionate Secularism to Indiscriminate Action represents a reframing towards an understanding more prepared to countenance coercive measures. Such a translation may occur under circumstances where a conflict of interests undermines the sustainability of unconditional support for people with HIV/AIDS. The case of the Public Sector Manager, described under the Indiscriminate Action heading above, seemed to approximate to this pattern: AIDS being 'detached' from equal opportunities concerns in order to avoid raising issues of sexual orientation. A, as yet, hypothetical instance where this type of translation could be applied is where Trust hospital managers perceive a competitive advantage by demonstrating that staff are 'HIV free'. If coupled to financial survival such a strategy, which would probably involve mandatory testing, could supplant 'pre-market' equal opportunities ideals.

The increasing spread of HIV among women might also be expected to elicit this type of transformation as (male) managers seek, consciously, to establish congruence between the treatment of women who are HIV positive and the generally inferior terms, conditions and benefits available to women workers in general (see Goss and Adam-Smith, 1995).

The Indiscriminate Action to Compassionate Secularism keying can be seen as a shift towards what is commonly regarded as ' good practice'. Such a move may be facilitated by access and/or exposure to education and training regarding HIV/AIDS: several of our Compassionate Secularism respondents cited such exposure as a critical incident in the development of their views on both AIDS and sexuality. Alternatively, the efforts of pressure groups may contribute to such a transformation – such attempts can be seen in the National AIDS Trust's 'Companies Act' and the Terrence Higgins Trust's 'Positive Management', both of which seek to demonstrate that good practice contributes to a creditable corporate reputation. It could be argued (see fabrication 1 below) that in some cases a fabrication is a necessary first step to securing the attention required to bring about this type of keying.

The keying from Compassionate Moralism to Punitive Moralism represents a shift from a position of tolerance to one of repression. Such a shift may be the result of an individual or group's perception that the objects of their pity and tolerance have failed to 'keep their side of the bargain' by, for example, refusing to defer to implicit rules of heterosexual normality or through defiant, and apparently 'uncaring', displays of 'difference'. One respondent expressed the following view illustrating this precarious balance:

> I mean I've seen incidents and read cases about them, there was a column in the Sunday paper a couple or weeks ago where this journalist was stuck on a train full of homosexuals and they were being discriminative against straight people and abusive. Nothing happened to them so why should anything happen to straight people if they are discriminative against them?

In Goffman's terms, the discreditable are, by their actions, discredited and thereby legitimately stigmatized.

In the reciprocal version of the previous keying, i.e. from Punitive Moralism to Compassionate Moralism, there is a revision of opinion allowing the 'reaccrediting' of a stigmatized individual. This is likely to take place on a particularistic basis such that the keyed frame applies only to one specific individual who, by their behaviour, has at least partially redeemed aspects of their spoilt identity. This is likely to be an unstable frame to the extent that it may revert to Punitive Moralism should the individual fail to maintain their 'acceptable' behaviour. In our data, this type of transformation was also used to differentiate between 'guilty' and 'innocent' AIDS sufferers. Thus, one respondent held a distinctly Punitive position regarding heterosexuals and drug users who transmitted HIV on the grounds that these were regarded as knowing the risks, whereas homosexuals were reframed into a Compassionate Moralism perspective on the grounds that most infection had occurred before the transmission routes of the virus were understood. Such a transformation applied to women with HIV, however, may also be hard to sustain – especially in strongly patriarchal environments – given the more obviously embodied nature of heterosexual difference (especially in the context of putative promiscuity) and the willingness to define female sexuality as essentially and irredeemably corrupting.

Fabrications

Whereas there is an assumption that keyings are achieved through the knowing participation (or at least passive acceptance) of those involved, 'fabrications' involve the possibility of deceit. Here one party will try to reframe the activity with the intention of 'deceiving' the other. In Goffman's (1975) terminology, the intention of a fabrication is to 'contain' those subject to it within the construction of meanings provided by fabricators, these meanings being a 'reworking' of a particular strip of activity. Fabrications can be of numerous types, direct and indirect (the latter involving one party convincing a second party of a particular view of a third party, which the latter can do little or nothing to affect), and range from the malevolent to the benign (i.e. where the fabrication is deemed to be 'in the best interests' of the 'dupe').

First, a framing of Compassionate Secularism can be fabricated to a frame that is more in keeping with Indiscriminate Action. Such a fabrication could conceivably be invoked where an actor, individually supportive of the rights of people with HIV, is able to 'conceal' equal opportunities motives, say, within a frame more acceptable to a 'hostile' audience. This may, in part, apply to the case of 'informal/hidden conflict' discussed above where issues of sexual identity are concealed within the less contentious notions of trust and cultural support. Another instance of this form of benign fabrication can be found in publications of a national AIDS charity: when addressed to 'sympathetic' organizations, AIDS is presented explicitly as an equal opportunities issue, but in a recent flyer for a conference aimed at 'less committed' business leaders, its significance is reframed, as the following extract from this flyer illustrates:

HIV AND AIDS COULD KILL YOUR MARKETS, YOUR PROFITS, YOUR ECONOMY AND YOUR PERSONNEL. $50 billion is the estimated cost of lost productivity, lost markets and retraining incurred last year by the world economy. HIV and AIDS predominantly affects the economically most important age group, 25–40 year olds – in the UK 90% of HIV positive men are between 20 and 49 years of age – the prime period when your managers, skilled workforce and most highly motivated staff yield their greatest return on your investment – and women are equally AT RISK.

(capitalization as in the original)

Second, an actor may try to fabricate a Compassionate Secularism frame from an Indiscriminate Action base. Such a transformation may arise when an individual, most probably a manager, wishes to maintain maximum flexibility of operation in practice, i.e. to have an understanding of a situation that allows him or her to act wholly pragmatically (rather than in line with some predetermined moral/ethical principle) while presenting a 'public stance' that emphasizes 'good practice' and a modicum of political correctness. Such fabrications do not appear to be uncommon in relation to gender-based equal opportunities policy (Collinson, 1991; Collinson *et al.*, 1990), suggesting that women employees affected by HIV cannot automatically expect better treatment than gay men. Clearly, researchers such as ourselves may also have been the targets of such a fabrication! (A detailed analysis of how this is achieved through the medium of written AIDS policy is given in Goss, 1995).

A third fabrication involves an ostensible shift from Compassionate Moralism to Punitive Moralism. Such a transformation is likely to be necessary in circumstances where an actor may feel threatened by 'loss of face' if he or she does not appear to comply with group norms framed in terms of Punitive Moralism. There was certainly a sense of existence of this type of fabrication in interviews with men working in a strongly masculine shop-floor environment where to express sympathy for someone with AIDS was to be equated with the discredited identity of a 'closet' homosexual (see Collinson, 1992).

A final fabrication, from Punitive Moralism to Compassionate Moralism, has much in common with the second fabrication above in terms of the attempt to create a 'politically correct' bias. This type of fabrication has been described to us by health educators, especially those working in organizations, when confronting the intransigence of deeply rooted prejudice against people with AIDS and its capacity to dissipate during the training session, only to re-emerge when back in the 'real world'.

Conclusions

The foregoing discussion has tried to demonstrate the complex and frequently contradictory ways in which attempts to understand the experience of HIV/AIDS within workplace settings will also draw upon existing discourses of organization sexuality. In many organizations, however, this sexual configuration, while omnipresent, is not openly acknowledged; on the contrary, Burrell (1984) points to a pressure in formal policy and practice towards the desexualization of many modern forms of organization. However, the early characterization of AIDS as the 'gay plague' has meant that it carries with it a constant reference of homosexuality (Watney, 1989; Weeks, 1991) such that where the formally desexualized discourses of organization encounter AIDS this threatens a resexualization – in Mellor and Schilling's (1993:422) words, a 'return of the repressed'. Attempts to contain this 'threat' may thus be expected from those charged with maintaining desexualization by, for example, (re)defining AIDS as an issue concerned *only* with health, or denying its relevance as a workplace issue. Such attempts at containment, though, will not necessarily be accepted by all organization members and, as such, may be denied, challenged, or supplanted by alternative definitions and practices. At the extremes, two responses are possible. On the one hand, addressing HIV/AIDS as a workplace issue may alert some organization members to the 'hidden' prejudice faced by homosexual employees and lead them to support claims for more effective recognition and protection of the rights of 'sexual minorities'. On the other hand, and in contrast, confronting HIV/AIDS may amplify others' latent or suppressed homophobia and lead to calls for additional repression of 'other'sexualities. What we have tried to establish through the vehicle of frame analysis is that these meanings are not fixed or immutable but are amenable to transformation and challenge. In this respect there remains an important transformative role for a critical organizational practice that works to move organizational opinion and practice in the direction of the former position, i.e. towards what Cockburn (1991) has termed a 'long agenda' for equal opportunities. This needs to ensure both adequate protection for people who are affected by HIV (e.g. through a comprehensive sickness policy) and to work to combat homophobia, sexism and racism. This is not to say that HIV/AIDS must be addressed *through* equal opportunities policy (this may, in fact be inappropriate, see Goss and Adam-Smith, 1995), but rather to suggest that an active and wide-ranging culture of equality of opportunity will provide the most effective back-drop against which any secular response to HIV/AIDS (e.g. as a 'simple' health issue) can be developed.

Notes

1   In this chapter the focus of attention will be upon male definitions of heterosexuality and male homosexuality. This is not to deny the increasingly important need to develop an understanding of the impact of AIDS on women in organizations informed by feminist/female constructions of sexuality. For a discussion of some of these issues within the context of employment see Goss and Adam-Smith 1995; Richardson, 1989; Scharfe and Toole, 1992; Squire, 1993; Wilton, 1992.

2   This data is taken from a study of 11 organizations, with an average of 10 employees per organization interviewed during 1993. The interviews lasted between half-an-hour and two hours, were tape recorded and transcribed in full. Wherever possible interviews in each organization covered senior managers, line managers, clerical and manual workers. The organizations studied were drawn from the manufacturing, health care, voluntary/charity, hospitality, and public sectors and were located across the UK, although predominantly in the south east. They ranged in size from six to 2000 employees.

3   Herek and Glunt's research labels the axes of the typology Pragmatism/Moralism and Coercion/Compassion and define their quadrants as follows:

> First, the Compassionate Secularism pattern characterizes the general stance of the American public health community and of the lesbian and gay male community: endorsement of such non-moralistic pragmatic policies as distribution of condoms and sterile needles, as well as opposition to coercive measures such as quarantine ... Second, a pattern of Compassionate Moralism ... is reflected in the official pronouncements of the Conference of Catholic Bishops: compassion is urged for people with AIDS, but education about condoms is rejected on moral grounds ... Third, Punitive Moralism, endorsement of coercive measures and rejection of non-moralistic pragmatic policies, is perhaps best exemplified in the US by spokespersons of conservative political and

> religious beliefs … Indiscriminate Action … may reflect an acquiescent response set [and] considerable ambivalence concerning AIDS: views of people with AIDS as both dangerous and deserving of compassion … containment as well as pragmatic education and prevention.
>
> (cited in Pollack 1992: 28)

The criteria we use to allocate cases to categories have been developed inductively from our data to reflect the specific focus on sexual identity in the workplace whilst retaining the sense of Herek and Glunt's original categories.

4　We are not yet in a position to comment confidently on the factors that may affect the distribution of cases in terms of organizational/occupational characteristics. It does seem, however, that respondents in the 'pragmatic' side of the typology are more likely to be in 'professional' or more senior managerial positions than those on the 'moral' side. Similarly, those in the Compassionate Secularism category were more likely to be employed in organizations that encouraged a strong formal commitment to equal opportunities.

References

BURNS, T. (1992) *Erving Goffman*, London: Routledge.

BURRELL, G. (1984) 'Sex and organizational analysis', *Organizational Studies*, **5**(2), 97–118.

COCKBURN, C. (1991) *In the Way of Women*, London: Macmillan.

COLLINSON, D. (1991) 'Poachers turned gamekeepers', *Human Resource Management Journal*, **1**(3), 58–76.

COLLINSON, D. (1992) *Managing the Shopfloor*, Berlin: de Gruyter.

COLLINSON, D., KNIGHTS, D. and COLLINSON, M. (1990) *Managing to Discriminate*, London: Routledge.

GOFFMAN, E. (1963) *Stigma*, Englewood Cliffs: Prentice Hall.

GOFFMAN, E. (1975) *Frame Analysis*, London: Penguin.

GOSS, D. (1995) 'Writing about AIDS: framing policy', *Scandinavian Journal of Management*.

GOSS, D. and ADAM-SMITH, D. (1995) *Organizing AIDS: Workplace and Organizational Responses to the Epidemic*, London: Taylor & Francis.

HEARN, J. and PARKIN, W. (1987) *Sex at Work: the Power and Paradox of Organization Sexuality*, Brighton: Wheatsheaf.

HEREK, G. and GLUNT, E. (1991) 'AIDS-related attitudes in the US', *Journal of Sex Research*, **28**(1) 91–123.

KOLB, D. and PUTNAM, J. (Eds) (1992) *Hidden Conflict in Organizations*, London: Sage.

MELLOR, P. and SCHILLING, C. (1993) 'Modernity, self-identity and the sequestration of death', *Sociology*, **27**(3), 411–32.

MILLS, A. and MURGATROYD, S. (1991) *Organizational Rules*, Buckingham: Open University Press.

POLLACK, M., PACHELER, G. and PIERRET, J. (Eds) *AIDS: A Problem for Sociological Research*, London: Sage.

RICHARDSON, D. (1989) *Women and the AIDS Crisis*, London: Pandora.

SCHARF, E. and TOOLE, S. (1992) 'HIV and the invisibility of women', *Feminist Studies*, 18(1), 64–7.

SMITHHURST, M. (1990) 'AIDS: Risks and discrimination', in ALMOND, B. (Ed.) *AIDS A Moral Issue*, Basingstoke: Macmillan.

SQUIRE, C. (Ed.) (1993) *Women and AIDS*, London: Routledge.

WATNEY, S. (1989) 'The subject of AIDS', in AGGLETON, P., HART, G. and DAVIES, P. (Eds) *AIDS: Social Representations, Social Practices*, Lewes: Falmer Press.

WEEKS, J. (1991) *Against Nature*, London: Rivers Oram Press.

WILTON, T. (1992) *Antibody Politic*, Cheltenham: New Clarion Press.

Chapter 6

Towards Effective Intervention: Evaluating HIV Prevention and Sexual Health Education Interventions[1]

Deirdre Fullerton, Janet Holland and Ann Oakley

> HIV/AIDS is the most serious infectious disease epidemic of modern times, worldwide in scope and devastating to individuals, communities, and ... countries most affected by it.
>
> (Kelly and Murphy, 1992: 582)

> The sense of urgency around the epidemic has been an overriding cause of failure to conduct proper outcome evaluations ...'
>
> (National Commission on AIDS, 1993: 7)

Effective and rigorous evaluation of social interventions in the HIV prevention and sexual health-education fields has often been dismissed as unethical, impractical, or both. The randomized controlled trial favoured in recent years by doctors and other health professionals in situations where there is uncertainty about whether a treatment or programme works is particularly unlikely to be used in the HIV prevention field. Randomized control requires allocating individuals to experimental and control groups, with the latter receiving no intervention. The perceived moral urgency of the HIV/AIDS epidemic and the ethical issues involved in denying high-risk groups any intervention which *may* be effective are particular problems for this method of evaluation. In this chapter we will discuss the findings from a survey and evaluation of studies of interventions in HIV prevention and sexual health education. We will provide an overview of the different approaches that have been employed in these fields, paying particular attention to the method of evaluation. We will discuss the problems and potential of randomized controlled trials, illustrated by those studies in our survey that have used the approach.

Interventions designed to prevent the transmission of HIV by reducing risk behaviours offer the only chance of limiting the spread of the epidemic. Modern medicine and molecular biology have had little impact on the spread of HIV. Although there have been some advances in secondary prevention and the treatment of opportunistic infections in the developed world, a successful vaccine is unlikely for some years (Cohen, 1993; Sittitrai *et al.* 1990). Even where effective therapies do exist for sexually transmitted diseases, their spread cannot be successfully contained by medical therapies alone; modes of infection are rooted in social mores and environmental factors related in complex ways to the biology of disease. Preventing the spread of such diseases calls for a detailed understanding of the determinants of risk-taking behaviour in different social groups, and demands that the construction of intervention strategies should be based on this understanding.

Evaluating Interventions

'Evaluation is the process that will enable us to learn from experience' (Turner *et al.*, 1989: 316). The Panel on the Evaluation of AIDS Interventions convened by the US National Research Council defines three types of evaluation: *formative, process,* and *outcome* evaluation (Coyle *et al.*, 1991). *Formative* evaluations involve small-scale efforts to identify issues and relevant strategies prior to, or independently of, designing and implementing programmes of intervention. *Process* evaluations study the ways in which services or interventions are delivered; they are designed to describe what goes on rather than to establish whether it works or not. Only the third type of evaluation, *outcome* evaluations, are designed in such a way that they can generate answers to questions about the effectiveness of particular interventions in changing specified outcomes.

While all three types of evaluation have their place in an adequate scientific response to HIV/AIDS prevention, it is essential not to confuse the contribution that can be made by the different types. Many evaluations claiming to provide data on outcomes are really exercises in monitoring or surveillance which make claims about the effects of interventions rather than establishing effectiveness. Historically, there has been some confusion between these two aspects of programme assessment (Aggleton and Moody, 1992). A common design involves obtaining baseline, pre-intervention data, and comparing these with a second wave of data collected post-intervention, in order to generate claims about the capacity of the intervention to alter relevant variables. Any intervention has to contend with the effects of 'background noise' all the other factors that are changing at the same time as the intervention is being implemented. But the use of designs that lack a control population and restrict inferences of effectiveness to the comparison of pre- and post-intervention measures makes it almost impossible to isolate the sound of the intervention at all. It is the very complexity and multiplicity of factors influencing health attitudes and behaviours that strengthens the case for properly designed randomized control trials (RCTs) with sufficiently large numbers as the only reliable way of establishing the effectiveness of different types of intervention.

RCTs offer a means of establishing the effectiveness of different approaches to a problem, largely through securing an equivalence between the social characteristics of experimental and control groups, distributing unknown factors capable of influencing outcome equally between study groups, and reducing the possibility of researcher bias (Chalmers *et al.,* 1983, 1989; Schwarz *et al.,* 1980; Silverman, 1980). These advantages are achieved by dividing a population into subsets of randomly selected samples, which, because of their method of assignment, should not be systematically different from one another. This method offers the best chance of any post-intervention outcome differences between the randomly selected groups being due to the effects of the intervention itself. While the most efficient approach statistically is to randomize individuals, in the behavioural field there is a preference for group randomization, in part because some of the interventions under test operate at the group or community level.

The primary condition for an RCT is uncertainty about the effectiveness of a particular intervention. If there is certainty, based on sound scientific evidence, then an RCT is both unnecessary and unethical. In the face of *un*certainty, an RCT is ethical, and, by extension, any other approach to assessing effectiveness that cannot, for design reasons, be expected to generate an answer becomes *un*ethical. What is ethical may not of course be possible for practical or political reasons. In the HIV/AIDS field, political opposition to zero treatment has been responsible for what is probably a higher incidence of trials with no 'no treatment' control group than in any other field, despite the fact that such a design contravenes the premise – of uncertain effect – on which the trial is based.

Methods Used in the Review of Evaluations of Interventions

Undertaking the review of HIV/AIDS health promotion and education interventions has involved five main stages of work: (1) identifying studies in the area through electronic searches, hand searches of relevant journals, checking references on articles collected, and contacts with people working in the field; (2) collecting reports of relevant studies; (3) classification of these studies using a set of review guidelines that we have generated; (4) entering information about the studies onto a specialized computer database; and (5) generating descriptions of the field and formal reviews from the computer database. The review has relied mainly on reports available in the English language, and the major focus is on HIV/AIDS prevention interventions, but since much of the education about HIV and AIDS for low risk groups, and especially young people, has been carried out within the general framework of personal or sex education, this broader area has also been included. Studies of interventions with high-risk groups were included for their potential to throw light on the effectiveness of different approaches to the prevention of HIV/AIDS in the population at large, bearing in the mind the distinction between low-risk groups as *communicational strategies* and as *risk* groups themselves (Wellings, 1992).

A basic aim of the review was the identification of methodologically sound studies. The classification scheme used covered descriptive information about the interventions and assessments of the quality of the study. The *descriptive* categories included details of the programme content, background discipline, theoretical orientation, social characteristics of the participants, intervention site, programme provider, length of programme and measurement tool(s) employed. *Quality assessment* categories included issues concerned with both design and analysis: the extent to which the aims and outcomes of the study were clearly defined, the replicability of the study, the type of control used, the sample size, the unit of allocation, number of units assigned to each condition, pre- and post-intervention information, whether attrition was discussed, and type of analysis carried out. Building on the systematic work of other reviewers in the health, education and social welfare fields (Biglan *et al.*, 1987; Loevinsohn, 1990; Schnaps *et al.*, 1981; Schwarz *et al.*, 1980), an evaluation of the methodological status of the studies was made with reference to a list of eight methodological qualities. These qualities were: (1) clear definition of aims; (2) a description of the intervention package and the design sufficiently detailed to allow replication by others; (3) inclusion of a randomly allocated control group or a control group equivalent on sociodemographic and outcome variables; (4) provision of data on numbers of subjects recruited to each condition; (5) provision of pre-intervention data for each condition; (6) provision of post-intervention data for each condition; (7) attrition rates reported for each condition; (8) findings reported for each outcome measure as described in the aims of the study.

A study with all of the attributes discussed above could be described as achieving a 'gold standard'. A smaller group of core criteria from the above list were selected in order to divide the studies into two broad groups: 'sound' and 'flawed'. Sound studies were those deemed to meet the four criteria of employing control groups, providing pre- and post-intervention data, and reporting on all outcomes. In view of the small number of gold standard studies that the reviewing process identified, it was decided not to restrict sound studies to those using randomized controls, but to include those where control groups/ subjects were demonstrated to be comparable to intervention groups/subjects pre-intervention on relevant sociodemographic and outcome variables.

Two reviewers with backgrounds in quantitative social science independently assessed each study. Any disagreements were discussed and resolved with a third reviewer. A final element in the reviewing process consisted of judging the effectiveness of the programme from the information provided in the published papers, and bearing in mind the attributes of quality referred to above. These reviewer assessments of effectiveness were then contrasted with those provided by the authors themselves.

Results of the Review

A total of 1210 studies were located in the review, of which 886 were found to have a specific focus on HIV/AIDS. Of the 886, hard copies were acquired for

Table 6.1 Outcome evaluations – percentage (numbers) displaying different 'quality' atttributes

	%	N
Aims stated clearly	100	68
Randomized controlled trial	41	28
Replicable intervention	72	49
Numbers recruited provided	85	58
Pre-intervention data provided	44	30
Attrition discussed	76	52
All outcomes discussed	76	52
Post-intervention data provided for all groups	65	44

Table 6.2 Outcome evaluations – percentage (numbers) of studies with 'quality' attributes and meeting 'core' methodological criteria

	%	N
All 8	15	10
7	16	11
6	15	10
5	25	17
4	12	8
3	15	10
2 or less	3	
Total	100	68
'Core' methodological criteria		
All 4	26	18
3	16	11
2	25	16
1 or 0	34	23
Total	100	68

815 studies. These were read and classified into reports of evaluations and other studies. There were 114 reports of evaluations including 73 outcome evaluations. The total of 73 studies included 5 linked pairs of reports describing the same studies. Separate outcome evaluations therefore totalled 68 (see Tables 6.1 and 6.2).

Which interventions work?

We compared the claims to effectiveness made by authors of studies with those derived from the review process, bearing in mind the need for methodological soundness as a base for establishing effectiveness. Tables 6.3 and 6.4 compare the effectiveness of the studies judged from both these viewpoints. Seven (39 per cent) of the methodologically sound studies were judged effective by authors (Table 6.3) and five (28 per cent) by reviewers (Table 6.4). Authors judged 32 per cent of the flawed studies effective (Table 6.3), compared with 6 per cent for reviewers (Table 6.4). The largest difference between authors and reviewers for the flawed studies was that 43 per cent were considered unclear by reviewers because of methodological problems and/or lack of necessary information (Table 6.4), but none by authors (Table 6.3). Overall, there was 54 per cent agreement between authors and reviewers on effectiveness, and in 9 per cent of cases some agreement as to effect; in 16 per cent of cases authors said the intervention was effective and the reviewers disagreed, and in 21 per cent of cases the reviewers judged the intervention to be unclear or ineffective when the authors' view was that it was partially effective.

Table 6.3 Quality of study by authors' assessment of effectiveness: all outcome evaluations

	Effective		Partially effective		Not effective		Unclear		Total	
	%	N	%	N	%	N	%	N	%	N
Sound	39	7	61	11	0	0	0	0	100	18
Flawed	32	16	60	30	8	4	0	0	100	50

Table 6.4 Quality of study by reviewers' assessment of effectiveness: all outcome evaluations

	Effective		Partially effective		Not effective		Unclear		Total	
	%	N	%	N	%	N	%	N	%	N
Sound	28	5	67	12	5	1	0	0	100	18
Flawed	6	3	40	20	8	4	43	23	100	50

Some examples of methodologically sound studies

Authors may be motivated to regard their interventions as effective, and indeed may be encouraged by the publication policies of journals to highlight success and play down results which suggest that the intervention was ineffective or even harmful. They may perhaps have more information upon which to base their judgements than that provided for the reviewers in their published articles, but if that is the case, we would argue that the information *should* be made available in the article. The difficulties of making adequate assessment of effectiveness should not preclude the effort, and the following description of selected examples of the methodologically sound studies in our review demonstrate the value of their approach in the range of effectiveness they report. Nine of the 18 methodologically sound studies involved interventions with young people and 9 reported interventions with adult high-risk groups. We give some examples of each here.

Hamalainen and Keinanen-Kiukaanniemi (1992) conducted a controlled study of the effect on HIV/AIDS knowledge and attitudes of one 45-minute lesson on safer sex and STDs, including HIV/AIDS, with 15-year-old school-children in 18 classes in 9 elementary schools in Oulu, Finland. There were three study groups consisting of six classes each: the experimental group who received the lesson and had data collected on attitudes and knowledge before and six weeks after the lesson; a control group for whom data were collected at the same time as for the experimental group; and a second control group for whom data were collected only once at the end of the study. An increase in knowledge following the lesson was demonstrated in the experimental group. Girls, but not boys, in the first control group also increased their knowledge between the two data collection periods. The lesson avoided ' authoritarian' approaches, used language that was familiar to young people, included demonstration of condom use, and encouraged open-ended discussion.

Ashworth *et al.* (1992), also tested the effectiveness of a single (1-hour) lesson comprising a video about HIV/AIDS and a discussion led by AIDS educators in changing students' knowledge using two suburban and two urban schools in Georgia, USA. Increased knowledge was demonstrated two weeks later among students who had been given the lesson.

A third controlled study in an educational setting was Wenger *et al.*'s (1992) trial of HIV antibody testing and AIDS education. This examined the impact on communication about HIV risk and sexual behaviour in American college students. Students attending the student health clinic who were interested in HIV education and testing were randomly assigned to three groups: education alone, education plus testing, and a control group. Those who were in the education plus testing group demonstrated increased communication with sexual partners about HIV risk six months later, but no differences were found in knowledge about AIDS, number of partners or condom use between the three groups.

Rotheram-Borus *et al.*, (1991) undertook a study with a group of runaway adolescents. The intervention and control groups were non-randomized: 78 runaways at one residential shelter given up to 30 HIV/AIDS sessions were compared with 67 runaways at a non-intervention shelter; sexual behaviours were assessed before the intervention and three and six months later. Although the shelters were non-randomized (and the reason for this was not explained by the authors), there were no statistically significant differences in socio-demograpic characteristics or sexual behaviour between the two groups of young people prior to the intervention. The HIV/AIDS sessions addressed general knowledge about HIV/AIDS, coping skills, access to health care and other resources, and individual barriers to safer sex. After the sessions young people reported more consistent condom use and less high-risk sexual behaviour.

In a study by DiClemente *et al.* (1989), the intervention consisted of three class periods of AIDS instruction with a newly developed curriculum employing information about the causes, treatment and prevention of AIDS and other sexually transmitted diseases. Three middle and three high schools in the San Francisco area participated. Classes within schools were allocated to receive the intervention or not. All students were pre-tested on AIDS knowledge and attitudes and they were followed up immediately after the three-day intervention. Those who had been exposed to the AIDS curriculum had more correct answers to knowledge questions about AIDS and were more accepting of classmates with AIDS/HIV. There were no behavioural assessments, and it was not known whether the apparent changes in the educated group were sustained over time.

Three studies provide examples of interventions in adult high-risk groups. Landis *et al.* (1992) examined two different approaches – 'patient' referral and 'provider' referral – notifying sex partners of HIV-infected individuals in three public health departments in North Carolina. Consenting HIV subjects were randomly assigned to the two experimental groups, and provider referral resulted in a significantly higher partner notification rate.

Kelly *et al.* (1989) tested the effectiveness of a behavioural intervention that included AIDS education, cognitive-behavioural self management and sexual assertion training and the affirmation of social supports, on the AIDS-related knowledge and risk practices of high-risk gay men in a US metropolitan area. Group sessions were led by a clinical psychologist to provide an evaluation of a community-based AIDS education programme aimed at gay and bisexual men. Participants were asked to complete self-reports on sexual behaviour and to keep a record of risk behaviour over a four-week period on forms provided by the researchers. In addition, each took part in a series of role-play exercises designed to assess assertiveness in potentially coercive risk situations. Participants were randomly assigned either to the experimental condition or to a waiting list control group. The intervention consisted of twelve weekly group sessions of 75–90 minutes each, led by two clinical psychologists and two project assistants. Intervention sessions covered information about AIDS and HIV transmission, risk reduction techniques, and the previous high-risk activities of the participants, with the group leaders attempting to identify strategies that would reduce risk in each situation, reporting back from participants on the success of these strategies, assertiveness, relationship skills and social support development. After the intervention, both the intervention and control groups underwent assessment procedures, and at this point the control group were offered the intervention. The intervention group underwent a follow-up assessment eight months later, but with no control group for comparison. The programme found reductions in the frequencies of risky behaviours in sexual practices and an increased use of refusal skills following the intervention. The findings are restricted to white gay/bisexual men, as a high attrition rate was noted among the ethnic minority men in the study.

A second study by Kelly and colleagues (1991) used opinion leaders to endorse HIV/AIDS risk reduction behaviour change among gay men in one intervention city and two comparison non-intervention cities in Mississipi and Louisiana. Persons reliably indentified as popular opinion leaders among gay men in a small city were recruited to serve as behaviour change endorsers to their peers. The opinion leaders acquired social skills for making these endorsements and complied in talking frequently with friends and acquaintances. Before and after the intervention, surveys were conducted of men patronizing gay clubs in the intervention city and in the two matched comparision cities. In the intervention city, the proportion of men who engaged in any unprotected anal intercourse in a two-month period decreased from 37 per cent to 28 per cent with a reduction from 27 per cent to 19 per cent for unprotected receptive anal intercourse. There was a 16 per cent increase in condom use during anal intercourse and an 18 per cent decrease in the proportion of men with more than one sexual partner. Little or no change was observed among men in the comparison cities over the same period of time.

In the following sections we describe some of the findings of the review in relation to work with young people and describe four interventions for drug users that employed randomized control methods.

Working with young people

Historically, most HIV prevention programs for adolescents have been developed without sufficient empirical information about the strategies that would be most effective in motivating health-promoting behaviour change.

(DiClemente, 1993a: 160)

Young people have emerged slowly as a risk group for HIV/AIDS. Early work suggested that encouraging the adoption and maintenance of low-risk behaviours among young people is not an easy task (DiClemente, 1993a). For example, while many young people are aware of the importance of condom use in preventing HIV infection, condom use is low and inconsistent in many samples (DiClemente, 1990; Hingson *et al.*, 1990), and informed teenagers do not necessarily adopt safe sex and drug practices (Reader *et al.*, 1988). The knowledge base of many young people in relation to the status and modes of transmission of HIV/AIDS is relatively high (Dusenbury *et al.*, 1991; Fife-Shaw and Breakwell, 1992), including in the UK, where it has been shown that most young people understand the major transmission routes (Memon, 1990). In the UK, and many parts of the USA, HIV/AIDS education is not part of the national curriculum. Where particular school-based education programmes are carried out, few have been adequately evaluated (Fetro, 1988). Evaluated studies demonstrate the impact of school-based HIV/AIDS education on attitudes and knowledge rather than behaviour (see, for example, CRP Incorporated, 1993; DiClemente *et al.*, 1989). There is little scientific evidence in general for the effectiveness of school-based education programmes in limiting health risk-taking behaviour among teenagers (see Lewis *et al.*, 1990 for a review).

Three of the process evaluations and 29 of the outcome evaluations identified in this review concerned HIV/AIDS interventions with young people. Five of these were discussed in the section on methodologically sound studies (Ashworth *et al.*, 1992; DiClimente *et al.*, 1989; Hamalainen and Keinanen-Kiukaanniemi, 1992; Rotheram-Borus *et al.*, 1991; and Wenger *et al.*, 1992).

Some of the lack of scientific evidence about means of effectively preventing HIV/AIDS transmission through educating young people to adopt safer sex practices is due to the limitation in programme implementation. However, some of it is also due to methodological limitations in the programmes that have been implemented, and particularly in the way in which these have been evaluated. Three particular problems are the lack of adequate control groups, small or unbalanced sample sizes, and the failure to take account of substantial and differential attrition between intervention and control groups. Lack of adequate discussion of these methodological issues in the literature is striking (see, for example, Boyer and Kegeles, 1991; Mantell and Schinke, 1990; Schinke *et al.*, 1992).

These problems mean that it is impossible to say whether some interesting interventions are likely to be effective or not. For example, the impact of an innovative theatre-based HIV-education programme for 13–19 year-olds is difficult to interpret due to the lack of a control group (Hillman *et al.*, 1991). Some interesting work looking at peer- compared with health-care-provider AIDS education for young women, found provider education to have an effect on knowledge of sex risk, and peer education on knowledge about injecting drug use; again, interpretation of these 'effects' is difficult due to the lack of a control group (Quirk *et al.*, 1993). A comparison with a sample of inner-city adolescents of three different approaches to AIDS education – education on its own, condom instruction and decision-making plus communication and assertiveness skills – was complicated by the lack of a control group, and additionally by small sample sizes (Kipke *et al.*, 1993).

Methodological problems bedevil interventions, which may consist of well-thought out and promising programmes; for example Shulkin *et al.* (1991) evaluated a peer-led AIDS education programme with San Diego university students in four classes, but the basis of assignment to intervention or control conditions was unclear, attrition was unbalanced between intervention and control groups (43 per cent versus 79 per cent), no pre-intervention information was given about the characteristics of the different groups, and analysis of programme impact was on the basis of individuals rather than classes as the unit of randomization. Self-selection into an intervention programme can also be a problem.

As can be seen from this rapid overview, methodological rigour is lacking in this area, but there are some lessons emerging from the studies and reviews that have been done on work with young people to which we would like to draw attention. It is important to listen to teenagers about their levels of knowledge, beliefs, understandings, and self-perceived needs, including in relation to sexual health in general (Miller and Moses, 1990). The social factors that lead to, and or support, behavioural change among teenagers must be identified, to form the basis for effective HIV/AIDS education programmes and intervention programmes, which need to be launched early in adolescence, before high-risk behaviour patterns are established (DiClemente, 1993b). Wider cultural issues related to taboos around sex and the empowerment of women must be also be addressed in the work (Holland *et al.*,1991; Wight, 1992).

In terms of the design of studies, an adequate period of follow-up is essential; for example Huszti *et al.* (1989) found that, while a comparison of lecture-based and video-based education with a control group showed better impact for the lecture-based method, knowledge scores for all three groups declined between the post-test (immediately following the intervention) and the one month follow-up. In terms of delivery, peer-assisted interventions appear to be effective (DiClemente, 1993b) as in the field of smoking prevention (see, for example, Telch *et al.*, 1990). The impact of intervention programmes may differ by gender (CRP Incorporated 1993); and by ethnicity (Aggleton, 1992; DiClemente, 1993a).

Much existing work adopts a negative definition of sexual health, equating it with the absence of STDs and the avoidance of unintended teenage pregnancy, rather than with the presence of qualities such as sexual pleasure and sexual enjoyment. It is important that programmes should include the 'positive' side of being young (Aggleton, 1992; Lewis *et al.*, 1990).

Lewis *et al.* (1990) argue for a move away from the traditional approach to school-based HIV prevention programmes in order to recognize the different bases of sexual and other risk-taking behaviour in this age group, and to take account of socially-rooted developmental processes. Theoretical understandings of the likely bases for risk-reduction behaviour need to take account of socialization processes, including young people's relationships to their families and peer cultures, and processes of generational differentiation.

Interventions for drug users

Four studies relating to drug users involved randomized control methods: Calsyn *et al* (1992), Des Jarlais *et al.* (1992), McCusker *et al.* (1992) and Baker *et al.* (1993). Calsyn *et al.* compared three conditions, with 313 injecting drug users seeking treatment in Seattle, Washington assigned randomly to each condition. The conditions were: (1) a 90-minute group AIDS education session; (2) the AIDS education session with optional HIV-antibody testing; and (3) a four-month waiting list. The AIDS education covered information about transmission, medical aspects of AIDS, and HIV-antibody testing and a three-tiered risk reduction strategy. Four months later the 218 users who could be located (the attrition rate was 30 per cent) were assessed for behavioural changes in a structured interview similar to the pretest interview. Like other investigators, the authors observed that the IDUs as a group were reducing their involvement in high-risk behaviours. But in contradiction to their hypothesis, they found no differential benefit from the AIDS education programme with a random assignment control group design. They point out that their findings concur with those of Gibson *et al.* (1991) and McCusker *et al.* (1992).

Des Jarlais *et al.* (1992) undertook a randomized trial of an AIDS prevention programme or a control group with no intervention for 104 heroin users whose main method of use was intranasal (snorting), and who had injected no more than 60 times in the previous two years. They were also hepatitis B negative. Assorted recruitment procedures were used and a payment of US $20 was made on completion of intake data collection, which consisted of a questionnaire covering drug use history, sexual behaviour and AIDS knowledge. A urine sample was taken for drug testing, and pre-test counselling was given and subjects asked to give a blood sample for HIV testing

(87 per cent agreed). The purpose of the programme was to prevent injection among those who had never injected, and further injection among those who had previously injected, by building up skills to this end, but safer injection techniques were included. A total of 83 subjects were located for follow-up between 5 and 21 months after intervention (20 per cent attrition) and asked about drug use and sexual behaviour since the intervention. The authors concluded that the intervention was effective in delaying the transition from sniffing to injecting, but a considerable amount of vital information was omitted from the write-up so that it is not clear in fact whether the intervention was effective.

The objectives of the McCusker *et al.* (1992) study were to compare the effects of two AIDS risk reduction interventions: (1) informational, based on 'standard' AIDS education programmes, consisting of two one-hour group sessions with a video, lectures, homework and class discussion; and (2) an enhanced intervention, based on social cognitive theory and relapse prevention theory and consisting of six one-hour groups sessions followed by a 30-minute individual health education consultation focused on personal susceptibility, situational analysis and skill building. The sessions used a range of methods involving experiential learning. As the two-session informational intervention was given either early (during the first week of a 21-day detoxification programme) or late (during the second week) there were three experimental conditions, and no non-intervention control group. A blocked randomization design with pretest and multiple post tests was used. The intervention periods were randomly ordered in blocks of three. Of the 567 clients who entered the treatment programme three-quarters attended all group sessions, the retention rate was lower for the enhanced condition (68 per cent). Immediately after the interventions, enhanced groups members reported significantly greater self-efficacy to talk themselves out of risky behaviour in relation to HIV transmission, but other knowledge and attitudes scales did not differ by intervention. At follow-up sessions, significant reductions in risky drug use were reported by all groups, and enhanced group members reported significantly greater reduction in injection frequency than did those in the late information session condition. But apart from frequency of injection, there were no significant differences in changes in behaviour between the intervention groups. The authors concluded that the informational intervention was moderately effective, there was no effect of the differences in timing of the intervention, and the relative effectiveness of the enhanced intervention versus the informational interventions was disappointing.

In the Baker *et al.* study (1992), 95 injecting drug users enrolled in methadone programmes in central Sydney were randomly allocated to three conditions: (1) a six-session relapse prevention programme; (2) a 60–90 minute individual motivational interview accompanied by a self-help manual;

and (3) a non-intervention control group. The hypothesis to be tested was that the Relapse Programme would be more effective in reducing risk taking behaviour than the brief intervention. All subjects were administered the Drug Use Scale and HIV Risk-Taking Behaviour Scale of the Opiate Treatment Index and had an HIV-antibody test at pre-intervention assessment and six month follow-up. At follow-up, answers to the Highest HIV Risk-Taking Behaviour Scale, collateral reports from subjects' sexual partners in relation to the previous month and urine analysis results for the month before follow-up were collected for 80/95 subjects (a retention rate of 84 per cent). There were no significant differences between groups in risk-taking behaviours during the month before follow-up; there was evidence of a lower rate of needle-risk behaviour (sharing and cleaning) during the heaviest risk-taking month since pre-intervention assessment in condition (1). There was no evidence that the brief intervention was of greater benefit than the usual methadone treatment, and neither intervention appeared to reduce sexual risk behaviour. The results are cautiously interpreted by the authors as showing that individual relapse prevention programmes decrease the level of needle-risk behaviour during relapse episodes, but that further research is required to replicate the finding.

An adequate research and evaluation design increases the confidence with which effectiveness of intervention can be assessed, and in these cases as we can see, the effectiveness was limited. In some cases behaviour change was reported for some activities, regardless of whether the individual was in the experimental or control group.

Conclusions

... the AIDS epidemic is a social as well as a biomedical phenomenon ...
From a social perspective, AIDS is, for the most part, a preventable disease that is inextricably rooted in the behaviours that transmit HIV.
(Miller and Moses, 1990: 39)

This review has found that only a small proportion of HIV/AIDS prevention interventions have been evaluated in such a way that it is possible to come to reliable conclusions about demonstrated effectiveness. The review has identi-fied a number of serious problems with such evaluations that dilute the potential of much existing work to offer useful clues as to the way forward in this field. While early in the epidemic the general lack of evaluation of prevention interventions reflected the moral emergency response to HIV/ AIDS, its persistence points to a more permanent and worrying problem in the dissonance between 'natural' and 'social' scientific approaches to knowl-edge. The findings reported in this review as to the methodological quality of

HIV/sexual health behavioural interventions fit with those in the health education field more generally. Claims to effectiveness in the health education field are considerably more common than hard evidence (Tones *et al.*, 1991).

Having noted these points, it is nonetheless possible to be clear about directions it would *not* be sensible, on the basis of existing evidence, for future work to take. First, the blunt instrument of mass media information and education has been shown not to have any demonstrated effect on behaviours relevant to HIV transmission (Darrow and Valdiserri, 1992). Second, conclusions about the effectiveness of prevention interventions in bringing about behavioural change must be limited to the small group of methodologically sound studies that have examined and reported on behavioural outcomes. Insofar as there is sound evidence of behavioural change from these studies, this is restricted in the main to well-educated middle-class white men in the USA, living in gay communities which have been particularly hard hit by AIDS (Kelly and Murphy, 1992).

In their 1992 paper on future directions for health promotion work relevant to HIV, Darrow and Valdiserri identify five principles on which this work should be based. These are: (1) that targeted messages for people at risk of acquiring or transmitting HIV should require their involvement and be based on appraisal of their current state with respect to stages of behavioural change; (2) that assessment of the effectiveness of interventions designed to change behaviours should be based on the ability of the intervention to move people with high risk behaviour to lower or no risk behaviours in incremental stages; (3) that the social and cultural contexts in which interventions are developed and evaluated should be analysed; (4) that HIV AIDS prevention should be integrated with STD prevention, drug-use education and education in family planning; and (5) that interventions should be evaluated for their ability to contribute to the overall goal of sexual health.

To these we would add that future interventions aimed at influencing behavioural factors relevant to HIV/AIDS transmission should be based on sound theoretical approaches; use appropriate quantitative and qualitative procedures and statistical techniques for analysing effectiveness; and where possible employ the design of randomized controlled trials.

Notes

1   This research was funded jointly by the Medical Research Council and the Health Education Authority. The research team was Deirdre Fullerton, Janet Holland, Ann Oakley, Sean Arnold, Deborah Hickey, Peter Kelley and Sheena McGrellis.

References

AGGLETON, P. (1992) 'Young people, HIV/AIDS and social research', *AIDS Care*, **4**(3), 243–4.

AGGLETON, P. and MOODY, D. (1992) 'Monitoring and evaluating HIV/AIDS health education and health promotion', in AGGLETON,P., YOUNG, A., MOODY, D., KAPILA, M. and PYE, M. (Eds) *Does it Work? Perspectives on the Evaluation of HIV/AIDS Health Promotion*, London: Health Education Authority.

ASHWORTH, C. S., DURANT, R., NEWMAN, C. and GAILLARD G. (1992) 'An evaluation of school-based AIDS/HIV education program for high school students', *Journal of Adolescent Health*, **13**, 582–8.

BAKER, A., HEATHER, N., WODAK, A., DIXON, J. and HOLT, P. (1993) 'Evaluation of a cognitive-behavioural intervention for HIV prevention among drug-users', *AIDS*, **7**(2), 247–56.

BIGLAN, A., SEVERSON, H., ARY, A., FALLER, C., GALLISON, C., THOMPSON, R., GLASGOW, R. and LICHTENSTEIN, E. (1987) 'Do smoking prevention programs really work? Attrition and the internal and external validity of an evaluation of a refusal skills training program', *Journal of Behavioural Medicine*, **10**, 159–71.

BOYER, C.B. and KEGELES, S.M. (1991) 'AIDS risk and prevention among adolescents', *Social Science and Medicine*, **33**(1), 11–23.

CALSYN, D., SAXON, A., FREEMAN, G. and WHITTAKER, S. (1992) 'Ineffectiveness of AIDS education and HIV antibody testing in reducing high risk behaviours among drug users', *American Journal of Public Health*, **82**(4), 573–5.

CHALMERS, I., ENKIN, M. and KEIRSE, M.J.N.C. (Eds) (1989) *Effective Care in Pregnancy and Childbirth*, Oxford: Oxford University Press.

CHALMERS, T. C., CELANO, P., SACKS, H.S. and Smith, H. (1983) 'Bias in treatment assignment in controlled clinical trials', *New England Journal of Medicine*, **309**, 1358–61.

COHEN, J. (1993) 'Sombre news from the AIDS front', *Science*, **260**, 1712–3.

COYLE, S.L., BORUCH, R.F. and TURNER, C.F. (1991) *Evaluating AIDS Prevention Programs*, Washington, DC: National Academy Press.

CRP INCORPORATED (1993) *AIDS: An Extensive Study*, Washington, DC: CRP Incorporated.

DARROW, W.W. and VALDISERRI, R.O. (1992) 'New directions for health promotion to prevent HIV infection and other STDs', in CURTIS, H. (Ed) *Promoting Sexual Health: Proceedings of the Second International Workshop on Prevention of Sexual transmission of HIV and other Sexually Transmitted Diseases*, Cambridge 24–27 March 1991, London: BMA.

DES JARLAIS, D.C., CASRIEL, C., FRIEDMAN, S. R. and ROSENBLUM, A. (1992) 'AIDS and the transition to illicit drug injection – results of a randomized trial prevention program', *British Journal of Addiction*, **87**, 493–8.

DICLEMENTE, R.J. (1990) 'Adolescents and AIDS: Current Research, Prevention Strategies and Public Policy', in TEMOSHOK, L. and BAUM, A. (Eds) *Psychosocial Perspectives on AIDS*, Hillsdale, N.J.: Lawrence Erlbaum.

DICLEMENTE, R J. (1993a) 'Confronting the challenge of AIDS among adolescents: directions for future research', *Journal of Adolescent Research*, **8**(2), 156–67.

DiClemente, R.J. (1993b) 'Preventing HIV/AIDS among adolescents: Schools as agents of behaviour change', *Journal of the American Medical Association*, 270(6), 760–2.

DiClemente, R.J., Pies, C.A., Stoller, E.J., Straits, C., Oliva, G.E., Haskin, J. and Rutherford, G.W. (1989) 'Evaluation of school-based AIDS education curricula in San Francisco', *Journal of Sex Research* 2, 188–98.

Dusenbury, L., Botvin, G.J., Baker, E. and Laurence, J. (1991) 'AIDS risk knowledge, attitudes, and behavioral intentions among multi-ethnic adolescents', *AIDS Education and Prevention*, 3, 367–75.

Fetro, J.V. (1988) 'Evaluation of AIDS education programs', in Quackenbush, M., Nelson, M., and Clark, K. (Eds) *The AIDS Challenge: Prevention Education for Young People*, Santa Cruz, CA: Network Publications.

Fife-Shaw, C.R. and Breakwell, G.M. (1992) 'Estimating sexual behaviour parameters in the light of AIDS: A review of recent UK studies of young people', *AIDS Care*, 4, 187–201.

Gibson, D.R., Lovelle-Drache, J., Young, M. and Sorensen, J.L. (1991) 'Does brief counselling reduce risk in IV drug users? Final results from a randomized clinical trial,' *Seventh International Conference on AIDS*, 2, 70.

Hamalainen, S. and Keinanen-Kiukaanniemi, S. (1992) 'A controlled study of the effects of one lesson on the knowledge and attitudes of schoolchildren concerning HIV and AIDS', *Health Education Journal*, 51, 135–9.

Hillman, E., Hovell, M.F., Williams, L., Hofstetter, R. and Burdyshaw, C. (1991) 'Pregnancy, STDs, and AIDS prevention: evaluation of new image teen theatre', *AIDS Education and Prevention*, 3, 328–40.

Hingson, R., Strunin, L. and Berlin, B. (1990) 'Acquired Immunodeficiency Syndrome Transmission: Changes in knowledge and behaviors among teenagers. Massachusetts Statewide Surveys, 1986–1988', *Pediatrics*, 85, 24–9.

Holland, J., Ramazanoglu, C., Scott, S., Sharpe, S. and Thomson, R. (1991) *Pressure, Resistance, Empowerment: Young women and the negotiation of safer sex*, WRAP Paper 6, London: The Tufnell Press.

Huszti, H., Clopton, J. and Mason, P. (1989) 'Acquired Immunodeficency Syndrome educational program: Effects on adolescents' knowledge and attitudes', *Pediatrics*, 84(6), 986–94.

Kelly, J.A. and Murphy, D.A. (1992) 'Psychological interventions with AIDS and HIV: prevention and treatment', *Journal of Consulting and Clinical Psychology*, 60(4), 576–86.

Kelly, J.A., St Lawrence, J.S., Hood, H.V. and Brasfield, T.L. (1989) 'Behavioral intervention to reduce AIDS risk activities', *Journal of Consulting and Clinical Psychology*, 57(1), 60–7.

Kelly, J.A., St Lawrence, J.S., Diaz, Y.E., Stevenson, L.Y., Hauth, A.C., Brasfield, T.L., Kalichman, S.C., Smith, J.E. and Andrew, M.E. (1991) 'HIV risk behavior reduction following intervention with key opinion leaders of population: An experimental analysis', *American Journal of Public Health*, 81, 168–71.

Kipke, M., Boyer, C.B. and Hein, K. (1993) 'An evaluation of an AIDS risk reduction education and skills training (ARREST) program', *Journal of Adolescent Health*, 14, 533–9.

Landis, S.E., Schoenbach, V.J., Weber D.J., Mittal, M., Krishan, B., Lewis, K. and Koch, G.G. (1992) 'Results of a randomized trial of partner notification in cases of HIV infection in North Carolina', *New England Journal of Medicine*, **326**, 101–6.

LEWIS, C., BATTISTICH, V. and SCHNAPS, E. (1990) 'School-based primary prevention: What is an effective program?', *New Directions for Child Development*, **50**, 35–59.

LOEVINSOHN, B.P. (1990) 'Health education interventions in developing countries: a methodological review of published articles', *International Journal of Epidemiology*, **4**, 788–94.

MANTELL, J.E. and SCHINKE, S.P. (1990) 'The crisis of AIDS for adolescents: The need for preventative risk reduction interventions', in ROBERTS, H. (Ed.) *Crisis Intervention Handbook*, New York: Springer.

MCCUSKER, J., STODDARD, A., ZAPKA, J., MORRISON, C., ZORN, M. and LEWIS, B. (1992) 'AIDS education for drug users: Evaluation of short term effectiveness', *American Journal of Public Health*, **84**(4), 533–9.

MEMON, A. (1990) 'Young people's knowledge, beliefs and attitudes about HIV/AIDS: A review of research', *Health Education Research*, **5**(3), 327–35.

MILLER, H.G. and MOSES, L.E. (Eds) (1990) *AIDS:The Second Decade*, Washington, DC: National Academy Press.

NATIONAL COMMISSION ON AIDS (1993) *Behavioral and Social Sciences and the HIV/AIDS Epidemic*, Washington, DC: NCA.

QUIRK, M., GODKIN, M. and SCHWENZFEIER, E. (1993) 'Evaluation of two AIDS prevention interventions for inner-city adolescent and young adult women', *American Journal of Preventive Medicine*, **9**(1), 21–6.

READER, E.G., CARTER, R.P. and CRAWFORD, A. (1988) 'AIDS – Knowledge, attitudes, and behaviour: A study with university students', *Health Education Journal*, **47**(4), 125–7.

ROTHERAM-BORUS, M.J., KOOPMAN, C., HAIGNERE, C. and DAVIES, M. (1991) 'Reducing HIV sexual risk behaviors among runaway adolescents', *Journal of the American Medical Association*, **266**, 1237–41.

SCHINKE, S.P., ORLANDI, M.A., FORGEY, M.A., RUGG, D.L. and DOUGLAS, K.A. (1992) 'Multicomponent, school-based strategies to prevent HIV infection and sexually transmitted diseases among adolescents: Theory and research into practice', *Research on Social Work Practice*, **2**(3), 364–79.

SCHNAPS, E., DE BARTOLO, R., MOSKOWITZ, J., PALLY, C.S. and CHURGIN, S. (1981) 'A review of 127 drug abuse prevention program evaluations', *Journal of Drug Issues*, **11**(1), 17–43.

SCHWARZ, D., FLAMANT, R. and LELLOUCH, J. (1980) *Clinical Trials*, London: Academic Press.

SHULKIN, J.J., MAYER, J.A., WESSEL, L.G. and DE MOOR, C. (1991) 'Effects of a peer-led AIDS intervention with university students', *Journal of American College Health*, **40**, 75–9.

SILVERMAN, W.A. (1980) *Human Experimentation: A Guided Step into the Unknown*, Oxford: Oxford Medical Publications.

SITTITRAI, W., BROWN, T. and STERNS, J. (1990) 'Opportunities for overcoming the continuing restraints to behaviour change and HIV risk reduction', *AIDS*, **4** (suppl 1), 269–76.

TELCH, M.J., MILLER, L.M., KILLEN, J.D., COOKE, S. and MACCOBY, N. (1990) 'Social influences approach to smoking prevention: The effects of videotape delivery with and without same-age peer leader participation', *Addictive Behavior*, **15**, 21–8.

TONES, K., TILFORD, S. and ROBINSON, Y. (1991) *Health Education: Effectiveness and Efficiency,* London: Chapman & Hall.

TURNER, C.F., MILLER, H.G. and MOSES, L.E. (1989) *AIDS: Sexual Behaviour and Intravenous Drug Use,* Washington, DC: National Academy Press.

WELLINGS, K. (1992) 'Assessing AIDS Prevention in the General Population', Report for the Concerted Action Assessment of AIDS/HIV Preventive Strategies, Lausanne, Switzerland, University Institute of Social and Preventive Medicine.

WENGER, N.S., GREENBERG, J.M., HILLBORNE, L.H., KUSSELING, F., MANTOGICH, M. and SHAPIRO, M. (1992) 'Effect of HIV antibody testing and AIDS education on communication about HIV risk and sexual behaviour: A randomized controlled trial in college students', *Annals of Internal Medicine,* **117**, 905–11.

WIGHT, D. (1992) 'Impediments to safer heterosexual sex: A review of research with young people', *AIDS Care,* **4**(1), 11–21.

Chapter 7

Communities, Governments and AIDS: Making Partnerships Work[1]

Dennis Altman

Ten years ago I attended the first International Conference on AIDS in Atlanta, and many of those attending the 1994 Xth International Conference on AIDS in Yokohama have become friends and colleagues over the past decade in our common fight against HIV/AIDS. Others who were friends, lovers, colleagues have died, and as always my pride is mingled with sadness at their loss. As a gay man, I live in a community where death has become commonplace, and where the stress of our losses is compounded by the ignorance and the hostility with which too many people still view us. As a political scientist, I seek to understand how these individual deaths and discrimination are shaped by larger economic and political forces. And as an Australian, a country which is part of the vast Asian/Pacific region, my greatest commitment is to expand the links and common purpose with co-workers across national and ideological boundaries.

Above all, I want to speak of those whose voices cannot be heard because they lack the resources to attend international conferences on AIDS. I cannot speak for young girls forced into the sex industry in Burma and Thailand, for the terrified refugees of Rwanda and Bosnia, for young people living on the streets in Rio de Janeiro and Bucharest, for the lesbians and gay men terrorized in Iran and Pakistan, for the Aboriginal people of my own country whose life expectancies are so much lower than those of the dominant population. But I can recall their presence, and remind us of our responsibility for those who, because of poverty, ignorance, persecution and neglect, are most affected by this epidemic.

I also speak with a deep commitment to the empowerment of those people and communities most affected by HIV/AIDS, above all of those who are HIV positive, and whose bravery in fighting the disease and its stigma is a constant inspiration. The idea of 'community' is a complex one, but I speak not in general terms but rather of those people who share a common sense of purpose and all too often a common oppression, whether this be based on their gender, race, sexuality or HIV status. Whether in Uganda or the United States of America, in Poland or the Philippines, it has been the affected communities that have taken the lead in mobilizing the political will and energies necessary to deal with the impact of this epidemic.

We need to distinguish between different epidemics, both in terms of epidemiology and resources. We know that in Asia, as in the rest of the developing world, AIDS will spread rapidly, primarily through unprotected heterosexual intercourse, and that both education and care will be enormously hampered by the inequitable division of resources between and within nations. We have all heard the rhetoric that only partnership between governments, health professionals and affected communities can meet this challenge.

Unfortunately, while governments are more powerful and have better resources than community organisations, they often lack the will to act effectively. An Indian Health Minister, for example, recently claimed that there is no fear of an AIDS epidemic in his country. AIDS demands both economic and political resources, and relatively few governments have been willing either to take effective and sometimes unpopular decisions or to work in genuine partnership with those groups most affected by HIV. At the same time, we need to recognize that neither the government nor the non-governmental organization (NGO) sectors is monolithic – there are divisions and possible alliances that cut across both sectors. In many cases the perseverance and courage of government officials has pushed governments into action when their masters would have preferred silence. Nor do all NGOs represent communities: some are created only to tap foreign donors, who too often support the well-written application rather than the messier reality of grassroots work.

Partnership

Meaningful partnership between government and communities implies common goals, but also mutual respect and adequate resources. Too often governments expect NGOs to rubber stamp their own programmes, and fail to accept that partners have different interests and priorities. Despite World Health Organisation (WHO) resolutions to provide funding to the non-government sector, too few governments are willing to enact this decision and make the funds available. Governments must avoid the temptation – not unknown in rich countries – to see the community sector as a source of cheap labour to disguise government inadequacies.

Governments can mobilize resources and commitment, can accept responsibility for basic care and support, and can do much to combat ignorance and discrimination. As the Director General of WHO, Dr Nakajima, said in speaking to heads of government:

> Your influence is great and by your personal commitment, you can do much to allay fear and prejudice. Set an example by visiting people affected by HIV/AIDS in their homes, hospitals and health centres; listen to them, and confront the reality of their needs, their sufferings and the difficulties they are going through.
>
> (WHO, 1994)

However, community-based organizations (CBOs) have certain real advantages. Ungphakorn and Sittitrai (1994) have identified three of these: flexibility; access to multidisciplinary skills; and most significant, the development of participatory programmes. The last advantage implies the empowerment of those affected, which means challenging the practice of most governments, who feel threatened by programmes that seek to give control over their own lives to women, to young people, to homosexuals, to sex workers, to injecting drug users, and to those perceived as dying of a fearful disease. We cannot hide the fact that the required empowerment and community development that this epidemic demands is subversive. To save lives, governments need to provide space and resources for unpopular and oppressed communities, and protect them against their critics.

Effective action to stop the spread of this epidemic, and to care for those already infected, is subversive because it disrupts existing power relationships. It is easier to organize another conference than to address the root causes of inequity, discrimination and poverty that underlie the rapid spread of HIV across so many parts of the world. As UNICEF (1993) has said:

> Containing the spread of the disease entails tackling deeply embedded traditions that encourage discrimination against young people (particularly young females), allow harmful cultural practices and preclude discussions of sexuality.

It is impossible to underestimate the importance of addressing the interconnected questions of gender inequality, sexual ignorance and exploitation, and widespread poverty and discrimination.

Let me give an example: too often, the necessary stress on heterosexual transmission of HIV in Asia is used to deny the existence of homosexual men, often at great risk of infection. The unwillingness of governments and health officials – indeed, of some NGOs – to acknowledge this, means that these men are denied access to the basic information and recognition that could help save their lives. Equally, many governments claim against all evidence that needle use and sex work are not a reality in their countries. In the face of HIV, such denial is the most effective way of encouraging the epidemic's further spread.

Success against AIDS demands an honest discussion of sexuality, gender, political and economic power, the global maldistribution of resources, and the monopoly of therapeutic drugs by a small number of powerful firms – honesty about all those obstacles that humans have created and thus have the power to change. International AIDS conferences and seminars must go beyond medicine to explore factors such as the systematic denigration of women in many countries, and the economic structures that deny many people with HIV-related illnesses access to simple and effective therapies. It is difficult for governments to be honest when this means drawing attention to realities unpalatable to powerful interests. Equally, CBOs must never lose sight of their role as advocates because of the immediate need for service delivery. Particularly in the rich world, too many CBOs have been co-opted by governments in return for resources, and are finding, perhaps too late, that in return they lose the capacity to speak for their community.

A Case Study

On balance, Australia offers an example of a successful decade of partnership between community, government and health professionals (Altman, 1992). I recognize that ours has been a comparatively easy path: Australia is a small and rich country, and we have had a succession of national health ministers committed to a partnership approach. This has meant government support for community-based initiatives and programmes working directly with people with AIDS, with gay men, with needle users, with sex workers, with people with haemophilia and with Aborigines and Torres Straight Islanders. Partnership has meant the provision of needle exchanges, of safe sex information, of support for home-based care programmes and, most important, a willingness on the part of government to listen to AIDS organizations and to include them in the development of policy.

But there are traps in partnership as well. Under pressure to cooperate with government, the community sector can replicate the institutions of the state, with its 'leaders' being increasingly unelected, unaccountable and unrepresentative – those who buy the logic of government are those who survive the system. Thus, despite the partnership, the Australian National Council on AIDS has become less representative of the communities most affected by AIDS. Our ability to resist government definitions of what is acceptable is constantly being tested, as the visionaries are replaced by the bureaucrats, the community leaders by the ambitious professionals and accountants.

Yet the fight against AIDS in Australia has produced some extraordinary alliances, friendships and mutual support. There are times when we join hands and tears in memory of those who have died, and I am reminded of the deep partnerships this disease has forged between unexpected allies. There have also been moments when the partnership has failed, and the interests of the most vulnerable and the most marginal are sacrificed to the short-term interests of governments or AIDS organizations.

At times, communities need to stay outside the governmental system – there is no doubt that ACT UP in the USA had more impact by doing this. While ACT UP's tactics may be inappropriate elsewhere, the basic lesson of retaining community independence and integrity is not. Once community organizations lose a process of open decision making and participatory involvement, they cease to be able to empower their constituents, and, however valuable their services, something essential is lost.

But is this concept of community empowerment too western a concept? And is advocating these principles a benign form of imperialism, as has been said at previous conferences of some of the interventions from ACT UP? These are legitimate questions, and I can only say that my own experience, and the testimony of others, suggests that the basic principles of the Ottawa Charter – which include 'empowering communities and assisting their ownership of their endeavours and destinies' – are valid in very different social, economic and cultural contexts. Just as HIV cares neither about race nor gender, so the need for voluntary and confidential testing, for humane care, for the provision of adequate information, is not limited by the religion or the economic system of any country.

Empowerment and Justice

In many countries, governments will talk privately to affected communities while ignoring them in public rhetoric. This is not good enough: visible recognition is important as a way of legitimizing community development and challenging social stigma. Even WHO has been timid too often in recognizing the leadership role taken by communities such as sex workers or gay men. As the President of the Western Australia AIDS Council said of this year's World AIDS Day theme of 'the family'.

> In its press release ... WHO identified feelings of trust, mutual support and shared destiny as essential constituents of a family. It specifically defined family to include street kids, sex workers, injecting drug users, religious associations and even the corner store, but could not bring itself to acknowledge the existence of gay families.

Too often, WHO and other agencies treat gays as does the American soap opera *Melrose Place* – both marginalizing and trivializing us.

Both justice and pragmatism demand that the voices of those most affected by HIV/AIDS be heard, and that their expertise and their right to human dignity be acknowledged. While governments persecute sex workers, injecting drug users and street kids, they merely compound their vulnerability to HIV. Thus, the tendency to view sex workers as 'vectors of infection', without any recognition of their very real oppression, is wrong, both morally and practically. Unless and until we recognize the central role of empowering people who are in the sex industry – in the vast majority of cases because of social and economic pressures – we will fail many of those who are most vulnerable.

The concept of cultural difference is often invoked to claim that programmes empowering sex workers or injecting drug users or street kids will not work. When this is said we need to ask: in whose favour does this argument work? Are there not Asian gays, African drug users, women forced into sex work in the Middle East and Europe? The voices of those, who claim 'cultural difference' makes frank discussion of sex or of drug use 'unacceptable', are too often the voices of those who would silence the poor and the weak in the interest of retaining their own power.

AIDS demands that we recognize the impact of political and economic systems, and identify governments and cultural institutions, that create barriers to effective prevention and care. There is a basic human right to dignity, to adequate information, and to appropriate care that transcends cultures and ideologies. To the extent that we are all vulnerable to the effects of poverty, torture and infection, human rights are indivisible. In the words of the UN Secretary General Butros Ghali:

> We must remember that forces of repression often cloak their wrongdoing in claims of exceptionalism. But the people themselves time and again make it clear that they seek and need universality. Human dignity within one's culture requires fundamental standards of universality across the lines of culture, faith and state.
>
> (Butros Ghali, 1993)

AIDS in Asia

The great revolutions this century in Asia against external colonialism and domestic repression should remind us that the assertion that human rights or political self-determination are somehow 'not Asian' is itself a reverse form of colonialist mentality that denies the history of the last century. AIDS demands *both* legal/political and socio/economic human rights: the rights to freedom of speech, organization and expression are central, but so too are rights to basic care and survival. This is not a case for western complacency: the impact of structural adjustment on many developing countries – and the misuse of resources by many governments – means that, however many HIV projects are put in place, they will merely be band-aids across the wounds created by economic injustice.

Partnership, too, applies to international agencies both governmental and non-governmental. It means the creation of genuine networks and coalitions across borders that has been the mandate of the International Council of AIDS Service Organisations (ICASO) and the Global Network of People Living with HIV/AIDS (GNP+) over the past few years. Yet, as we in the community sector have struggled to build genuine networks from the bottom up, we find that too many agencies would rather pay consultants to discover what is already known than provide infrastructure for existing community groups. There is a growing industry of well-paid advisers making flying visits to 'the field' – while in some agencies you have to fill out three forms to buy a worker a cup of coffee or mail a letter. While ICASO, GNP+, etc. are fragile and incomplete networks, they are the closest to representing those most affected at a global level. Far better support them than to embark on the creation of yet more international organizations.

Research partnerships too are crucial, as in the extraordinary role that community groups have played in biomedical AIDS research, already beginning to impact on other diseases (Epstein, 1995). One of the achievements in my own country was the early development of sophisticated collaborative research between academics and the gay community, in ways which have helped us develop effective educational interventions (Kippax *et al.*, 1993). These examples suggest that researchers need show more humility in the face of the enormous knowledge and experience of community workers (Altman, 1994). As Jonathan Mann has said:

> Each affected community, each community responding to AIDS, is a laboratory of discovery in HIV/AIDS prevention and care. The capacity for accelerated global learning among communities is central to progress against AIDS, just as international sharing of scientific information from different research centres is fundamental to scientific advance.
>
> (Mann, 1993)

We need more economic, social and political analysis, but such analysis poses threats to government control and hence is dangerous. AIDS is not primarily a matter of individual behaviour and responsibility, but rather a disease of poverty, discrimination and ignorance, which requires an analysis based on political economy not more studies of knowledge, attitudes and behaviour. This may require a total rethinking of the organization of future international conferences on AIDS, to get away from the apparent division of the necessary knowledge about the epidemic into four self-contained tracks.

Partnership means a sense of common purpose and respect for divergent tactics: too often we attack our allies while leaving the real enemies – ignorance, intolerance, gross inequalities – to go unscathed. The spread of HIV is hastened both by the distortion of government resources into military spending and grandiose development projects, and by denial and ignorance in the name of tradition and religion. With HIV it is no longer possible to believe that Papal pronouncements against condoms or Hindu and Islamic prohibitions of homosexuality are 'merely' questions of personal values or traditional beliefs; people will live or die depending on how far traditional prejudices and superstitions are allowed to survive. The rhetoric of taking responsibility for one's actions, so often applied to those with AIDS, must be applied to religion, government and business – religious inflexibility is as guilty of killing people as is the tobacco industry.

If this sounds harsh, remember the devastation of this disease – in the cities of Newark and Paris; in the villages of Uganda and India; in the slums of Bangkok and Port au Prince. As Elizabeth Reid wrote:

> One story from the Kagera region in Tanzania is of a young girl sitting day after day at the edge of the yard, rocking on her heels and staring into space. Both her parents are dead, brothers and sisters, aunts and uncles. There is little food but she is not hungry. She rocks, grieving.
>
> (Reid, 1992)

I remember today a young man from Goa who was incarcerated because he was HIV positive, and on his release fought discrimination against those with HIV in India until his death. Dominic de Souza was young and fragile, but he spoke with such moral strength that senior officials exerted great efforts to keep him from the stage at international meetings. Dominic played a key role in the establishment of the Asia/Pacific network of community organizations, and he showed us that a sense of community embraces all those who are prepared to accept the realities of human diversity and fight against the realities of bigotry, injustice and inequality. From him, and thousands like him, we can draw both the resolve to build real partnerships, and the strength to speak the truth, however politically inconvenient or embarrassing it may be.

NOTES

1   This chapter was first presented as a plenary address at the Xth International Conference on AIDS in Yokohama.

References

ALTMAN, D. (1992) 'The most political of diseases', in TINEWELL, E. *et al.* (Eds) *AIDS In Australia*, Sydney: Prentice Hall.

ALTMAN, D. (1994) *Power and Community: Organisational and Cultural Responses to AIDS*, London: Taylor & Francis.

BUTROS GHALI, B. (1993) 'Democracy, development and human rights for all', *International Herald Tribune*, June 10.

EPSTEIN, S. (1995) The Construction of Lay Expertise: AIDS Activism and the Forging of Credibility in the Reform of Clinical Trials', *Science, Technology and Human Values*, **20**, 4.

KIPPAX, S., CONNELL, R.W., DOWSETT, G.W. and CRAWFORD J. (1993) *Sustaining Safe Sex: Gay Communities Respond to AIDS*, London: Taylor and Francis.

MANN J. (1993) 'A global epidemic out of control?', *AIDS Asia*, December 5.

REID, E. (1992) *The HIV epidemic and development: The unfolding of the epidemic*, New York: UNDP.

UNGPHAKORN, J. and SITTITRAI, W. (1994) 'The Thai response to the HIV epidemic, *AIDS*, **8** (suppl. 2), S155–163.

UNICEF (1993) *AIDS: The Second Decade: A Focus on Youth and Women*, New York: UNICEF.

WORLD HEALTH ORGANISATION (1994) Press Release *WHO/46*, Geneva: WHO.

Chapter 8

Socially Apart Youth: Priorities for HIV Prevention

Ana Filgueiras

This chapter offers a preliminary analysis of the particular vulnerability to HIV infection of millions of children and young people who are out of, or beyond the reach of, formal schooling. It adopts a global perspective, examining the experience of what might be described as 'socially apart youth', a term that is used to remind us of the primary factor that exposes relatively distinct groups of young people to HIV infection. Street kids, children in difficult circumstances, marginalized youth, and many other expressions do not underline the common denominator among these young people. They are all outside the social system and lacking access to services and information. Whether a refugee, an abused child, a young person on the streets, or an adolescent in institutional care, these are children who are denied the human rights so eloquently described by Jonathan Mann and others (GAPC, 1993). Three main issues are examined: what health and health promotion means for socially apart young people; what it means to be young in developing countries; and how can we achieve the biggest possible impact at all levels reaching different youth communities as much as each unique child or adolescent.

Health is perhaps best viewed in terms of each person's ability to defend against environmental, social and personal threats. Common environmental threats to socially apart youth include cold weather and pollution, common social threats include violence, civil strife, and discrimination, and common personal threats include forced and unsafe sex, preventable diseases, and malnutrition. Health promotion is the process through which people achieve physical, mental and social well-being. It is above all the ability each person has to use resources on a sustainable and equitable basis. It involves the ability to identify needs, look for resources, and cope with constraints – accessing clean water, food, and a safe place to sleep, getting information about health prevention measures, and to seeking and obtaining treatment.

In relation to young people, health and health promotion means challenging several adult assumptions. Central among these is what is youth? Just like adults, young people are not a homogenous group. This is often said, but practice shows that many adults still tend to view all young people as inherently irresponsible, rebellious, and risk-taking, always in a permanent search for immediate pleasure. With such an attitude we are ultimately placing on young people themselves the responsibility of an eventual HIV infection. But in many cultures and within specific constraints young people might be exposed to risk or protected because of adult pressure, an over-protective family, or religious beliefs. They might be exposed to HIV infection because their parents sell them into prostitution, forced early marriage, or the care of silently abusive house masters.

Although not homogenous, young people share some factors in common. They are people still in a process of development through specific cognitive stages. An understanding of the different abilities and difficulties within the distinct stages of development is crucial in order to help young people develop and adopt skills to cope positively with their daily life. Additionally, and despite a diversity of cultures and socio-economic situations, all adolescents experience the passage into adulthood. They must all learn to cope with physical changes, get used to emergent sexual desire, and with the changes associated with puberty. Adolescence is always a period of life in which a re-examination and exploration of feelings, desires, possibilities, limits, social and gender role expectations occurs.

As young people experience life, including sex, adults ask themselves if adolescents should know about sex. Instead of assessing what their practices are and what kind of information they might need, adults frequently deny young people access to adequate information. Recently, the World Health Organisation examined 19 studies conducted in Australia, Europe, Thailand, and the United States of America to assess the impact of sex education on the sexual behaviour of young people. The conclusions showed that sex education does not promote or increase sexual activity, but in some cases may in fact encourage young people to delay penetrative sex, to reduce the number of sexual partners, or to have safer sex (Baldo *et al.*, 1993). Ultimately, by refusing to provide accurate information and skills, adults leave young people exposed to abuse, unwanted sex, or sex early in life. Rather than question when young people should or should not be sexually active, we would better use our time to ask them what they want to discuss and be informed about, so that they can be accurately informed in order to adopt safer practices.

The same occurs when people ask themselves if condoms should be available to young people. The question that we must ask not ourselves but young people *themselves* is what information they need, and where this needs to be provided. Young people will not stop being sexually active simply because of a lack of condoms. They will continue to exercise their sexuality, but in an unsafe and unprotected manner. Of course, merely distributing condoms is not sufficient, and we must also talk openly about other forms of safer sex, including abstinence, masturbation, and non-penetrative sex.

Yet how can we take into account the wide range of young people's views and experiences? How can we ensure a proper approach to meeting their health needs? In what ways do young people define health and illness? And are the answers to these questions the same as those that would be given by the youth workers running programmes? What are young people's priorities; how can we best find out these things; what makes socially apart youth distinct; and what factors add to their vulnerability?

Socially apart young people are often those living in poverty with little or no access to even the most basic social and health services. They have no money to pay for transportation to get to school or to pay school fees. They are overwhelmed early in life by hard work and other responsibilities in order to help support the family. Homelessness is common and can be due to civil conflict and unrest, famine, or because families fall apart. Street children running away from poverty or domestic abuse, young people orphaned through AIDS, or migration are other distinguishing factors. Many drop out or are truant from school because educational programmes and curricula ignore their culture, stage of development, or discriminate against their ethnic or religious backgrounds. Families often find it difficult to cope with a child's substance use. They lack the skills necessary to deal with the problem and understand the dynamics behind the use of substances in the first place, or they may not have the necessary support to cope with their own problems. The situation can become so bad that the young person leaves home.

Whatever the reason, vulnerability is increased because socially apart young people are exposed to adult exploitation, including that of the sex trade. Violence, the use of multiple drugs to cope with physical and emotional pain, stress caused by fatigue, fear, a lack of self-esteem, ill health including untreated sexually transmitted diseases, the list of risk factors for HIV is very long.

Gender Inequality and AIDS

One-third of people living with HIV are women, and more than half are under the age of 25. At the Xth International Conference on AIDS in Yokohama, Michael Merson, Director of WHO's Global Programme on AIDS, pointed out that up to 60 per cent of all infections in females occur by the age of 20. Other studies have shown that in sub-Saharan Africa, 60 per cent of new infections are among people between the ages of 15 and 24 years, and that of these more women than men are HIV seropositive. Young women between the ages of 15 and 19 years are four times more likely to be HIV infected than their male counterparts.

Gender inequality means that there are fewer opportunities and less power for women to avoid unsafe sex or negotiate for safer sex. There is evidence that women are pushed to become sexually active at an earlier age than men, and that they tend on average to become infected by HIV many years before young men. Older men in many countries, called 'sugar daddies' in some cultures, are now seeking out young women for sex in the belief that these girls are less likely to be infected with HIV. This is happening all over the world, but especially where AIDS is having a visible impact.

Pregnancy and STD rates among young women are high and reflect the potential exposure to HIV through unprotected sexual intercourse. In some countries in Africa, one-third of all teenage girls become pregnant before the age of 17 years. Every year 5 million abortions occur among women between the ages of 15 and 19 years, many of them illegal, a factor which for most women results in unsafe and life-threatening conditions. One in 20 teenagers worldwide is estimated to have a sexually transmitted disease, although the actual figures are probably much higher but difficult to calculate because young women have difficulty recognizing symptoms, or else they do not seek treatment because in many settings treatment is equated with the stigmatization of being sexually active. Also, in an attempt to avoid pregnancy, or for reasons of pleasure, anal intercourse is commonly practised.

Young women's vulnerability to HIV infection is also higher because of the physical trauma caused by sex at an early age. Female genital mutilation, as part of traditional rites in many African and Arab countries, is another practice that increases the physiological risk of infection. Between 85 and 114 million women have suffered genital mutilation worldwide, usually performed when they were at the age of 4–8 years old. Women who have suffered genital mutilation are often forced to engage in anal sex while vaginal intercourse is not possible, thus adding to their vulnerability to HIV infection.

Pregnancy and childbearing is a major factor forcing young women to drop out of school, depriving them of the education and skills needed to gain employment, and often leaving little choice but to sell sex for survival. Young women are deprived of the same educational opportunities often because their parents lack the economic means to pay school fees, or else their attendance at school is not seen as important compared with men due to social norms. The traditional status and role of women means that they are expected to carry the burden of domestic tasks and care for the family.

Poverty and miserable living conditions deprive young girls of even minimal privacy, exposing them to the risk of sexual assault and rape – often by family members where incest is one of the most accepted or silent abuses either within the family or community. Girls who have their first sexual experience through rape are often socially outcast and rejected by the family and community. In many cases these young women leave home to escape such abuse or to avoid depriving the family of the breadwinner or mother's companion. Homeless and without any means of social support, these young women become subjected to the potential risk of HIV infection while living on the street.

Gay and Lesbian Youth

Too often young people in developing or developed countries are pushed out of their homes, their communities, or even their countries because of their sexual preference, or because they are searching for their sexual identity. They are discriminated against and abused in schools with the silent complicity of teachers until they drop out of school. They are humiliated and ignored in programmes traditionally devoted to working with young people by the constant denial or lack of understanding of youth workers. They are sexually abused by adults working in penal institutions, refugee camps, or in war areas. This lack of awareness, understanding, and support for gay youth forces many to be socially apart.

We must implement innovative programmes that seek to understand and take into account issues that until now have been constantly denied or ignored by those working with young people in developing countries. These include programmes that are sensitive and non-judgemental, and which are rooted in the needs of gay and lesbian youth. This requires a brave stance against the widespread but false notion that people make a choice about their sexuality, and that in the case of young people they can be influenced or manipulated to adopt one lifestyle or another. In fact, anyone who has ever really listened to a young gay person will be convinced that sexual preferences are not about choice. The youth worker's role should not be one of trying to convince young people what is right or wrong, but of respecting their rights to live and be as they are. Only when we learn to accept and respect sexual and social diversity can we hope to make progress against the spread of HIV.

Empowerment for Prevention

The concept of empowerment is often used without a full appreciation of its meaning and importance. Empowerment involves supporting a person's ability to cope with constraints, such as discrimination on any basis such as race, gender, religious affiliation or sexual identity. It is the support one must have in order to manipulate social mechanisms for the defence of individual and social rights.

In the case of young people, this notion must be specifically redefined, especially when, as socially apart youth, they are deprived of any family or community support. For these children and adolescents to develop their potential fully, empowerment must be viewed as a means of creating a supportive environment that allows them to express their needs, desires, pleasures or pains and the other full range of emotions necessary for the growth of self-esteem. The development of young people is dynamic and evolving, with some limitations, yet boundless possibilities.

To offer an example, sometimes young people who are HIV positive are encouraged to be open about their antibody status, despite the possibility that they may be living in a discriminatory and abusive environment. In other occasions, a young sexually abused girl may be told that it is appropriate to speak out against her abuser, even though protective measures to ensure her safety and well-being can not be guaranteed. Street children in Brazil have been shot at by the police because, with the backing of outreach workers, they dared to point out police corruption and torture to the press. Because of this, we must never encourage young people to confront their oppression and abuse when there are insufficient measures to ensure their safety and survival. Without these guarantees, the concept of empowerment becomes nothing more than a cruel and empty promise, and sometimes an abusive action.

We must push hard for the provision of legal advocacy, especially in developing countries where large numbers of young people are denied their primary human rights such as lack of access to existing goods and services necessary for the development of their overall well-being, including education and health services. Such advocacy initially designated to support the defence of individual and social rights can be most effective in opening pathways to clinical, educational, and welfare services when available, but blocked by the bureaucratic or discriminatory net that places young people socially apart from existing services.

We urgently need to provide and reinforce joint programmes in solidarity between non-governmental organizations and international agencies. Education, prevention, and care must be planned and provided in an integrated way. Programmes should be expanded in a way that mobilizes society as a whole. The Red Ribbon campaign offers a good example of a simple, cheap, and effective tool for increasing AIDS awareness. The health system must have safeguards to protect against discrimination towards the poor, young people, and ethnic and religious minorities. Researchers must be mobilized, and we must learn how to use their findings and their data to advocate for concrete responses to the needs of young people. And we must find ways to define, advocate and respond to a common agenda on human rights, where abusive practices and behaviours can be definitively abolished.

Antigone Hodgkins, the executive director of a youth run organization called Bay Area Young Positives in San Francisco, has convincingly reminded us that any educational strategy addressing socially apart youth must be designed, planned, and implemented with the active participation of the young people themselves. It must be developed and evaluated stage by stage, step by step, as close to young people as possible and incorporating their opinions and perspectives. Besides needing specific support, HIV-positive young people need to be involved in programmes and services to guarantee quality and relevance. However, young people must not be used to merely legitimize the ideas and agendas of adults. The tokenistic involvement of youth in programmes and services is offensive and counterproductive. Instead, we must support young people by developing their skills in communication and negotiation so that they can participate fully and as equals. Again, we must never create a situation where they are made to feel responsible or guilty for their HIV serostatus.

I will conclude this chapter by reiterating two points. Children and adolescents, like other human beings, are unique as individuals, each child and each adolescent establishes and develops different relationships with their peers, their family, their community, and their environment. That is why our biggest challenge is to be able to design programmes and services in such a way that they will have a positive effect on the promotion of health within a specific youth community, while being meaningful to each unique child, adolescent, and young adult within that same community.

Out of school youth, children in difficult circumstances, street kids, children who are refugees, or socially apart youth, whatever label we give them, the common denominator is that they are young people. They have needs, desires, and dreams as children in any culture and in any part of the world. Like all children they need to be loved and listened to. They need us to leave behind our preconceived ideas and prejudices, and to approach them and their problems on their level as individuals. They need our trust, without the moral judgement that will inhibit them and lock their fears inside. To ensure this, we must provide a safer and more supportive environment.

References

BALDO, M., AGGLETON, P.J. and SLUTKIN, G. (1993) 'Does sex education lead to earlier or increased sexual activity in youth?', poster presentation (D02 3444) at the IXth International Conference on AIDS, Berlin.
GAPC (1993) *Towards a New Health Strategy for AIDS*, Boston, MA: Global AIDS Policy Coalition.

Chapter 9

Theorizing and Researching 'Risk': Notes on the Social Relations of Risk in Heroin Users' Lifestyles

Tim Rhodes

There is a four letter word that has gained enormous popularity in the AIDS era. Not only does it punctuate almost every conference paper and journal publication on the subject of HIV and AIDS, it litters the talk of interventionists, policy makers and researchers. If ever there was a 'keyword' that can be considered core to the study of the social aspects of AIDS, it is this word.[1] Look no further than the cover of this book or the title of this chapter.

Among those of us involved in HIV work, the word 'risk' has become something of a staple diet that feeds our thinking about intervention and research design as much as it influences our actions in the bedroom. It is the unifying theme that has helped to mobilize a disparate collection of disciplines within the 'scientific community' to do something about HIV and AIDS. The idea of risk seems as commonplace in contemporary sociological discourses as it does in Department of Health advertising campaigns. While on the one hand it is viewed as a unifying concept to identify, define and organize analyses of 'post' and 'late' modern industrialized societies (Adams, 1995; Beck, 1992; Giddens, 1991), it is also the conceptual bread and butter of HIV and drug prevention initiatives. Yet within the domain of HIV prevention and research, the notion of risk is little understood. It has barely even been questioned.

This chapter is an initial attempt to question what we mean by risk and its derivative epidemiological concepts of 'risk behaviour' and 'risk factors'. It briefly plots the key features of contemporary theorizing on risk and risk behaviour, and it explores the utility of some of these ideas for understanding risk and safety in the context of the everyday lives of heroin users. The aim is to examine how risk is best conceptualized in future research on the social aspects of AIDS. The method of doing this is to explore some preliminary findings from a qualitative research project that investigated the everyday drug taking and sexual lifestyles of opiate and stimulant users.[2]

Theorizing Risk: Epidemiological Constructions of Social Life

It has been the job of epidemiology to identify the determinants and distribution of HIV disease. This has been achieved by the defining, categorizing and monitoring of 'risk factors', 'risk groups' and 'risk behaviours'. It is within the parameters of risk defined by epidemiological research that lay and professional understandings about HIV infection and AIDS have emerged (Berridge, 1992). Epidemiological categorizations of risk factors and of risk groups have laid the foundations for the formation of targeting and intervention strategies adopted by prevention initiatives (Kane and Mason, 1992). This is both necessary and inevitable in the prevention of epidemic disease, but an unquestioned reliance on epidemiological definitions of risk is also short-sighted.

Epidemiological constructions of risk have encouraged a myopic vision of the social aspects of HIV risk and of lifestyles affected by HIV and AIDS. There is an inevitability about epidemiology doing this, for this is not unusual and pre-dates HIV disease. It is important to question, however, the power invested in such approaches and their utility in making sense of a complex social problem in a complex social world. The everyday lives and lifestyles of those affected by HIV and AIDS have largely been reduced, for the sake of study and of intervention, to measurable units that fall under the generic category called risk behaviour. This is the antithesis of the thinking that underpins our research, which aims to describe the social worlds in which people live as they describe and view them (Rhodes *et al.*, 1995). If epidemiology is concerned with reducing behaviour to neatly sized, easily manipulated units or variables of risk, then by contrast sociology and anthropology is concerned with exploratory descriptions of how risk is lived through interaction and experience. It is argued here that contemporary epidemiological thinking about HIV-risk is devoid of understanding about 'lived experience'.

This myopic vision characterizing epidemiological notions of risk behaviour has had direct implications for how HIV-risk has been conceptualized. It has encouraged a distorted picture of what people's lives are like and of where the risk of HIV infection fits in. It has little (if no) appreciation of the everyday lifestyles of populations affected by HIV and AIDS, or of how these lifestyles shape, mediate or influence perceptions of HIV-risk. It has been largely unable to envisage how perceptions of HIV-risk are contextualized by the mundane or bizarre of how and why people actually behave as they do. In short, when investigating risk from the perspectives of participants themselves (be these daily heroin injectors or weekend ecstasy users) epidemiological constructions of risk have a quality that is more imagined than real.

Yet in this chapter I am making no claims to knowing the 'truth' about risk. All that is being said is that it is often the case that epidemiological constructions of risk are taken as read, as known to be true, as objective and factual. At the very least these 'truths' should be questioned. This is the role of qualitative research on the social aspects of AIDS. As noted by Stephanie Kane, this has meant 'filling-in and questioning the empty categories of epidemiological prediction' (Kane, 1991: 1037). For others, it has meant untangling the ways in which responses to the HIV epidemic have been socially constructed as part of the 'invention' of AIDS (Patton, 1990). It is thus important to question the role and power of epidemiological notions of risk in constructing the 'HIV problem' as we know it today.

The fundamental limitation of current theories of risk, upon which conventional research notions are based, is associated with the concept of individual rationality. The bulk of HIV-prevention responses, be these syringe exchanges or safer sex campaigns, are based on theories of health behaviour that view risk perception and behaviour change to be the product of individual cognitive rational decision-making (Friedman *et al.*, 1994; Rhodes *et al.*, forthcoming). The key behavioural models or theories of health-beliefs (Becker, 1974), social learning (Bandura, 1977) and reasoned action (Fishbein and Azjen, 1975) theorize 'risk taking' to be the result of an individual's rational decision making based on the perceived costs and benefits of risk-related action. At their crudest, these theories assume a *single* rationality of risk perception and associated choice making. At their currently most advanced, these theories propose that risk perception and choice making is the product of a *situated* rationality, where rationality is inextricably linked to the specific contexts and situations in which risk-related action takes place. The key tenets of current theorizing on risk are summarized below. This then allows us to explore their utility in understanding risk as it is viewed and experienced by heroin users in the context of their social lifestyles.

Single Rationality Theories of Risk

Single rationality theories of risk assume that individuals' calculations and assessments of risk acceptability and susceptibility are rooted in a single rationality of what is healthy or harmful (Douglas, 1992). Individual actions to avoid risk are viewed as the 'healthy choices', calculated on the basis of rational decision-making about the probability and severity of potential harm. Risk avoidance (e.g. not sharing syringes) is synonymous with 'reasoned action' and is thus an exemplification of rational rather than irrational behaviour. Because such theories do not permit risky actions to be rational choices, even if based on adequate knowledge and beliefs about the actual probability and severity of harm, continued risk behaviour among drug users can often be viewed as the product of unreasoned or 'irrational' choice making.

Situated Rationality Theories of Risk

Without acceptance of anything more than a *single* rationality of risk perception and risk-related action, risky behaviour is relegated to the dubious categories of cognitive malfunction and behavioural dysfunction. It is for this reason, that *situated* rationality theories of risk posit that individual rationality is context and situation dependent. The costs and benefits of risk-related actions are influenced by contextual factors, which may have less to do with the calculation of scientific probabilities of risk and harm than with the calculation of *social* costs and benefits associated with acting in certain ways. Qualitative research has shown, for example, that some HIV-negative drug users continue to have unsafe sex with their HIV-positive sexual partners despite adequate knowledge of their personal susceptibility to HIV transmission (Rhodes and Quirk, 1995). While single rationality theories would conceptualize this as being a problem of individual perception and decision-making (much of lay and professional opinion would categorize such behaviour as 'irrational'), situated rationality theories conceptualize that such action is a product of *rational* decision making based on situation specific costs and benefits associated with unsafe sex (e.g. where loss of trust or intimacy between partners is perceived to be of greater cost than the risk of HIV transmission). What is perceived to be a cost, a benefit, or a risk is not static or necessarily shared among all individuals alike – be they drug users or epidemiologists – but is situated within different social contexts of belief and behaviour.

This gives insight into one of the key limitations of *any* theory of risk or change based on the concept of individual rationality. That rationality about risk perception and action is a *situated* phenomenon highlights that differential perceptions of risk and rational behaviour can exist. This underlines the fact that risk perception is socially organized. Risks are not simply or only 'calculated' by individuals, and neither is risk-related action necessarily individually 'chosen' or 'decided' upon. The costs and benefits of actions are socially organized because individuals' own thinking and behaviour is influenced by what is socially acceptable and legitimate. In the same way as everyday modes of injecting behaviour may be structured by specific group norms and values, individual risk perceptions are mediated by social norms about what risk is. Theories of *cognition* remain trapped within the heads of individuals; they are unable to discover how individual risk-related actions gain meaning through the everyday process of social interaction with others. As noted by Mary Douglas on the subject of risk perception:

> If a group of individuals ignore some manifest risks, it must be because their social network encourages them to do so. Their social interaction presumably does a large part of the perceptual coding on risks
>
> (Douglas, 1986: 67)

While situated rationality theories of risk recognize a plurality of *rationalities*, and are thus a significant improvement on single rationality theories, they nonetheless tend to reduce action to a product of *individual* decision or choice-making. This ignores the fact that what is considered risk (be this the probability of harm from HIV, HBV, overdose, or loss of friendship) varies by social situation and social network norms. What is often assumed to be a case of individual choice making is often not a product of individual choice at all. Such actions are not merely 'individual' or autonomous choices because they are often constrained or influenced by group social norms. Neither are they simply 'choices' because individual cognitive and behavioural actions are often constrained by a variety of exogenous social, cultural and economic factors (e.g. unsafe sex for money, or rape).

Social Action Theories of Risk

This exposes the misguided faith that most health promotion campaigns have in the concept of 'choice'. Presumed to be something made by individuals, choice assumes that risks are systematically *calculated* by individuals. This is not necessarily the case. Many behaviours in which drug users engage are seen by health professionals to be risky, although to drug users themselves they may be seen as nothing more than mundane everyday occurrences. The scoring and using of drugs is an obvious example. Because risk-related perceptions and actions are socially organized (in part by different networks or sub-cultures) they are also socially 'calculated'. This is why Mary Douglas has observed that it is social interaction (and not merely individuals) that 'does a large part of the perceptual coding on risks'. The fallacies of individual rationality and individual choice help to blur the fact that risk-related action is often a product of socialized *habituation* rather than calculation (Bloor, 1995). It is misleading, therefore, to view risk behaviour as 'risk taking' since this rather naïvely reduces risk-related action to nothing more than individual agency or mind set. Risk reduction clearly demands more than the tweaking of cognitive thought processes; it also requires changes in community norms and social structure.

Risk theory thus needs to account for the social organization of risk perception and behaviour. It needs to move beyond the restrictions of existing theories that view 'risk perception as an individual and not as a social phenomenon' (Douglas, 1986). As we are again reminded by Mary Douglas, dominant social scientific approaches to the study of risk – be these the dangers of exhaust emissions from the petrol in your car or of other environmental pollutants – have been noted for their inability to recognize the importance of *social* as well as individual actions: 'It seems that the neglect of culture is so systematic and so entrenched that nothing less than a large upheaval in the social sciences would bring about a change' (Douglas, 1986: 1).

Researching Risk: The Everyday Social Context of Heroin Users' Lifestyles

As we noted above, an investigation of risk and risk perception as a socially organized phenomenon is an advance on most research designs, which tend to restrict analyses to measures of risk behaviour as they are epidemiologically defined. While epidemiological research is ostensibly concerned with monitoring *what* trends in HIV-related 'risk behaviour' occur among drug users, it is largely unable to fully explain or predict *why* or *how* people behave as they do (Rhodes *et al.*, forthcoming). In investigating the production of HIV-related risk behaviour in the social context of heroin users' lifestyles, it is fundamentally necessary to describe how 'HIV-risk' is understood and experienced from the perspectives of heroin users themselves. This can be considered the first step to exploring the relevance, utility and appropriateness of epidemiological constructions of 'risk'. It is also a step towards describing the social lives of heroin users in terms of the rites, rituals, chaos and boredom of 'lived experience' rather than in terms of the technological order and predictability of dominant scientific constructs of 'HIV-risky lifestyle'.

There are two key tenets that inform our approach to research (Rhodes and Quirk, 1995). The first is to describe the *social meanings* attached by actors (in this case heroin users) to behaviours categorized as risky (and non-risky) by the health epidemiologist. Behaviours attributed risky by the epidemiologist are thus to the qualitative sociologist part of a wider structure or culture of behaviours and associated meanings, which to participants themselves are often viewed and experienced as 'normal', rational, even mundane (Schwartz and Jacobs, 1979). This means untangling 'the meaningful dimension' of the lives of heroin users, which, as pointed out by the anthropologist Margaret Connors, 'so far has been hidden behind an externally-constructed pastiche of risk behaviours only specific to AIDS' (Connors, 1992: 591).

The second tenet of our research approach aims to understand the *social processes* by which actors come to attach meaning to behaviours deemed risky by health epidemiologists. Rooted within an interactionist frame, this research aims to investigate how the meanings that actors attach to certain behaviours are produced through interaction itself. The meaning of injecting drug use as defined by most HIV-related epidemiology and health promotion is decontexulized from the meanings of these behaviours for actors. Only by investigating behaviour as an interactive process is it possible to glean how interaction gives such behaviour a 'meaningful dimension'. In other words, to understand the social meanings of certain risk behaviours for actors themselves, it is necessary to understand how risk is a situated phenomenon. We know enough about what researchers call risk; we need to know more about what risk means for the people who partake in such research. We need to understand the 'reciprocal effects of social settings upon individuals and of individuals upon social settings' (Schwartz and Jacobs, 1979: 9), rather than simply reducing the actualities of individual social lives to variables that offer the potential for statistical manipulation.

The importance of these points can be shown by discussing two examples drawn from recent ethnographic work undertaken in London (Rhodes and Quirk, 1995). Approximately one hundred drug users participated in the study, of whom two-thirds were primary users of heroin or other opiates at the time of interview. Findings indicated that there are a range of risks which heroin users perceived to be associated with the use and/or injection of drugs. These are shown in Figure 9.1.

As a means to examining the social aspects of AIDS, this chapter focuses on what has been epidemiologically constructed as *the* risk behaviour associated with heroin use: injecting drug use. If 'Silence=Death' can be seen as an icon or symbol of activist aesthetics associated with the cultural deconstruction and fight against AIDS (Patton, 1990), then 'Injection=Infection' can perhaps be seen to symbolize recent dominant social constructions of risk associated with heroin use. In popular representations of the heroin user, it is 'injection' that has been taken to signify what it *means* to use heroin (whether or not it is injected). Similarly, in HIV discourses it is the association of 'injection' with 'infection' that has served to mobilize the rationale and actions of scientific and prevention responses (as epitomized by national media campaigns: 'It just takes one prick to give you AIDS'). The meaning of injection for the epidemiologist and for health promotion *is* the risk of infection: it is little else, whether or not there are other risks, dangers or costs associated with this particular mode of ingesting a drug.

The social world of heroin use, therefore, has been reduced to a vision encapsulated by associations of injection with HIV infection. The epidemiological and prevention emphasis on HIV risks associated with injection have served to blur the social meanings of injecting as they are lived and experienced in everyday interactions by drug users themselves. This picture of what heroin lifestyles are about is not only bad news for HIV-related research, but is particularly bad news for HIV prevention. In the absence of a sensible

---

Addiction/Dependency
'This is a habit, you know, that's just gone on too long and it's really pissing me off'
'If I don't have any sort of opiate I don't feel well and I can't function properly'

Overdose
If you're injecting then obviously it's quite dangerous 'cos you could quite easily overdose'
'I mean basically if you overdose you die, you know, assuming you go right over'

Injecting damage
'I couldn't wear T shirts or anything, it was pissing me off ... all the scars and bruises'
'It's inevitable I'm gonna end up losing an arm or a leg and I don't wanna do that'

Sharing equipment
'I got hepatitis B through sharing ... I never done it since'
'blood poisoning, hepatitis, HIV ... I don't like the idea of anything going under my skin'

Using bad gear
'Buying bum gear ... you could kill yourself or give yourself a very nasty death'
'I'm just so dubious about street gear and what's in it'

Chasing/smoking
'I started chasing the dragon and eventually it ends up chasing you'
'I'm booting, can't be doing my lungs any good, my chest, it messes around with your body'

Buying and dealing
'We're really careful when we leave [dealers] sort of make sure we stash it somewhere'
'The only way you can get it [money] is by ripping someone off'

Other risks/dangers
'Most of my money goes on drugs'
'I was nicked last year for burglary'
'It takes over . . . I mean even like eating properly'
'Your sex drive in both male and female is virtually non-existent'

Figure 9.1 Risks associated with everyday heroin use

understanding of what risk and injection mean to heroin users themselves there is little chance of understanding how the 'HIV risks' associated with injection are prioritorized or acted upon. As argued in this chapter, HIV risks associated with injection are *relative* risks. This also means they are *situated* risks. They are perceived in the context of other risks, costs, benefits and meanings associated with the injection of drugs.

The qualitative data presented below focuses on injecting drug use. As is clear from Figure 9.1, other examples could well have been chosen to show how research on HIV risk has constructed a pastiche of 'risky lifestyles' associated with heroin use. The example of 'addiction' itself immediately springs to mind. The example of violence associated with the dealing of drugs might have proved another incisive case study, as might the risks associated with drug-related crime. By focusing specifically on injecting, a behaviour explicitly deemed 'HIV-risky', it becomes possible to clearly demonstrate how such a behaviour is seen, by drug users themselves, to carry a number of other (non-HIV) risks and dangers on a day-to-day basis. This helps give a better sense of what '*HIV* risk' means in people's lives and of why and how people behave as they do.

The aim of this chapter is not to further entrench ideas that injecting is the *only* risk in heroin users' lives. Neither does it aim to encourage a vision of heroin use that is *necessarily* characterized by risk. It is vitally important that the data presented below on the risks associated with injecting are seen in the context of other 'risks' associated with drug using lifestyles (see Figure 9.1). It is equally important to recognize that, on the whole, heroin users' lifestyles are not *intrinsically* risky. While it is necessary to focus on risk and injecting so as to examine the social relations of HIV-risk, heroin users' lifestlyes are not as racy or risky as the data presented in this chapter might suggest. Any readers unfamiliar with the world of heroin use should remind themselves, as they read the remainder of this chapter, that the lives of heroin users, perhaps on occasions like theirs, are more often characterized by boredom and doing nothing, than they are by personal danger or risky behaviour.

Overdose: 'Risk Priorities'

The first case example is overdose. Drug users' perceptions of HIV risks are part and parcel of a hierarchy of 'risk priorities' associated with injecting a drug. Findings showed that, on a day-to-day basis, the risk of overdose was perceived by many heroin injectors to be of greater concern than the risk of HIV transmission. The risk of overdose was an everyday concern; it was a *routinized* danger of injecting street heroin. Rather than being an unusual occurrence, the risk of overdose was seen to be an 'obvious' consequence of injecting: 'if you're injecting then obviously it's quite dangerous 'cos you could quite easily overdose'. Overdose was thus viewed as a 'great risk' and by some as the '*main* risk' associated with injecting:

> I think my main risk is overdose. That's my main risk because we did overdose the other day because as I say we got some really clean gear and we wasn't used to gear being that clean [because] we got used to the shit that we were taking
>
> (Male heroin injector)

The relative immediacy of perceived overdose risk is a function of the likelihood of overdose occurring. As one user responded in answer to the question 'Have you ever come near going over at all?': 'Yeah! Cor bloody hell, yeah!'. She went on to say: 'There ain't no one that I know that whacks[3] that ain't never gone over. There ain't no one that I know'. The immediacy of perceived risk is also a function of the immediacy with which overdose occurs:

> He got three score bags and I had a whack and the other two people had a whack and it was xxxx's whack right, and he's whacked up and, you know, sometimes people sort of sit down after they've had a whack and they'll gouch[4] like ... but he didn't, he just went smack on the floor. He was standing up and his last words were 'Fucking hell, I can feel that coming on' and he's just gone bang, bang on the floor, works[5] still in his arm. I was screaming 'Get an ambulance, get an ambulance!' and everyone was going 'No, no, no, he's alright' but he weren't ...
>
> (Female heroin injector)

The relative importance given to the dangers of overdose is a function of the likelihood of death occurring as a consequence. As noted by a male heroin chaser:[6] 'I realised when I did try a fix of gear that it was very strong and I could quite easily kill myself that way'. For some, overdose related deaths were not seen to be bizarre or unusual events but 'an everyday thing':

> Death is like a normal thing, like an everyday thing. If you take heroin you can be dead at any moment and it's not very frightening – you live with that. So it doesn't frighten you much like it would a normal person ... It was normal that even best friends, they died. I mean, it was sad, but it was normal, nothing special ... and I think that's why drug users are not so afraid to get AIDS
>
> (Female heroin chaser)

Death, and overdose-related deaths in particular, clearly have a different *meaning* for heroin users than for non-users or other 'outsiders'. Fatal overdose situations were described by heroin users with a degree of detachment that might not usually be the case when a friend or acquaintance dies on the sofa beside you. While users would often attempt to prevent death occurring when someone they know has gone over ('I stuck the fucker in the bath, poured cold water on him, he still didn't wake up. Finally brought him round'), this was not always the case. Indeed, some of the fatal overdose situations described were characterized less by action than they were inaction: 'I just couldn't bring him round so I just left. I just thought "Fuck it, if he dies, he dies".'

The normality of overdose deaths in some injectors' lives not only impinges on perceptions of 'risk priority' associated with injecting drug use, it also shapes perceptions of 'risk acceptability'. What is acceptable or legitimate action in response to a potential fatality occurring may carry with it different social meanings in the context of heroin use and overdose than in other contexts unrelated to drug use. Because overdose can be normalized or routinized as part of everyday heroin use it is also to some extent legitimized. Overdose falls within the boundaries of 'acceptable risks' associated with the injection of heroin. Ignoring the fact that somebody in the same room as you may be about to die from an overdose was thus considered, by some users, to be acceptable – or at least not unusual – behaviour. While this was by no means the case for all heroin users, there are two main reasons why *some* users felt that there were greater benefits associated with ignoring others' overdoses. The first was the perceived dangers associated with police interest when calling medical assistance:

> The best thing you can do is just to leave them. I mean, it's not very nice but you're not going to end up in prison cos some silly fucker's overdosed
>
> (Male heroin chaser)

The second was associated with not wanting to interrupt the 'buzz' from having taken heroin. One user explained that when having taken heroin 'you feel good' and 'you sit down and relax' because 'you've just been feeling rough'. In this context another's overdose is 'really annoying' and 'really' demanding'. As another user reported of a friend of hers whose partner died of an overdose:

> She jacked him up and he died and she just left him . . . she just went to bed . . . and said 'I knew what had happened but I just couldn't be bothered to do anything or ring an ambulance' . . . She said 'I was enjoying my buzz, didn't want to ruin my buzz' . . .
>
> (Female heroin injector)

That the everyday risks associated with overdose may be given greater priority by drug injectors than HIV risks highlights the importance of an interplay of factors associated with the ways in which risk is perceived. Perceptions of risk susceptibility and acceptability can be seen to be a function of the perceived *immediacy* of risk. HIV-related risk, when viewed in the social context in which it is perceived, is a *relative* concern.

Vein Damage: Situated Costs and Benefits

The boundaries or limits that regulate risk perception and action differ for different people. For some heroin users, the very act of injecting operated as a 'risk boundary'. The onwards transition from non-injecting use to injecting was taken to have specific symbolic meaning for heroin users who perceived such action as risky or 'really dodgy'. It was taken by some to be a signifier of 'dilapidation', 'deterioration', 'serious addiction' and 'junkie behaviour' often associated with increased personal and health costs. As was noted by non-injectors, 'people really fuck their bodies up through it', they have 'horrible ulcers and revolting arms' because 'all their veins are buggered up'.

But the injection of drugs was clearly also associated with certain benefits. These were largely associated with the immediate 'rush' or the 'better high' gained from intravenous injection. One other key benefit identified with injecting rather than chasing or snorting heroin was that injecting is more economical: 'definitely it's stronger to fix up and, you know, I could use less'. But for others, the costs associated with injecting were seen to outweigh the benefits. While injecting was seen as an indication of 'serious addiction', chasing or snorting was seen as a way of staying on 'stalemate road' and of preventing 'going in too deep'. Chasing or snorting was thus viewed by non-injectors as one way of minimizing the increased risks of addiction associated with heroin use ('it's easier to come off chasing'), as well as minimizing the risks of vein damage associated with frequent injections. As one user who had made the 'reverse transition' from injecting to chasing commented, chasing was seen to be 'safer':

> I was injecting and decided like, you know, it was too much messing around, messed up all my veins and that, so I started chasing.
>
> (Male heroin chaser)

Vein damage, like overdose, was often given a higher 'risk priority' than HIV as far as injecting was concerned. This was because such damage, and its consequences, were perceived to be more likely and immediate. Vein damage was seen to have two consequences for the successful injection of drugs, both of which can be seen to carry costs as well as benefits. The first is the risk of increased difficulty in having a hit or of losing the hit altogether. The success of locating and successfully hitting an over-used or deteriorated vein is often limited and can take some time, if not a lot of patience. Users, for example, talked of having 'their fifteenth attempt to get to some vein'. As described by one injector:

> [injecting] could take a couple of hours, and in the process I might lose my drugs, you know, because of needle clots or whatever, and blood gets into it (the syringe) and you can't use it ... Nevertheless I used to put myself through that constantly and as I say I literally have to spend between one and two hours trying to find, trying to get it into my system.
>
> (Male heroin injector)

As explained by other users, with damaged veins it is only possible to 'get a little bit in at a time so it can go off in the works and it'd be no good':

> If I tried to whack up I wouldn't get a vein it would clog up with blood, the works, the syringe, would clog up with blood and that's it, you wouldn't be able to use it, so you go with nothing. So rather than go with nothing you'd go for a boot.[7]

(Female heroin chaser)

For this interviewee, the difficulties in finding and hitting a vein and the risk of losing a hit encouraged a move back to chasing: 'my geezer turned round to me and said "Right, that's it, you ain't doing that no more, that's disgusting, you gotta go back to booting".' The relative costs associated with booting ('it won't do nothing, I wanna whack') were thus perceived to be the lesser of two evils in comparison with the costs of continued injection. For others, the risks of losing a hit through blood clogging in the syringe were avoided in other ways: by squirting the hit into the mouth when unsuccessful in finding or hitting a vein; by injecting non-intravenously ('skin-popping' or 'flesh-popping'); and by injecting elsewhere (where non-damaged veins still existed). A user describes a recent occasion where he witnessed a 'lost hit' being squirted into the mouth. His description shows that the risks of losing the hit were given greater priority than the risks of HIV transmission:

> He's got about half a gram, fifty quid's worth of gear in a syringe. Now he's trying to get a hit right, and he where he couldn't, where he's so, he'd had loads anyway and he's fucked up and like he was trying to get a vein and it was all clogging in the works. He goes "Ah, fuck it, I'm going to squirt that away, it's all clogged up with blood". Two people paid him a fiver each and had half of it squirted down their mouths with all his congealed blood in and everything. They took it orally, like, you know, just to save it being thrown away.

(Male heroin chaser)

As noted above, for those that did not make the reverse transition to chasing or snorting heroin, the second consequence of deterioration of veins was the need to inject elsewhere. When all available veins were depleted, this meant either considering injecting non-intravenously (skin-popping) or considering injecting into veins in 'riskier areas' of the body. Users saw there to be costs and benefits associated with both. While skin-popping can be seen to be one way of avoiding further vein damage, 'you don't get the rush' which, for one male injector, was seen to 'be quite bizarre' because 'you have to wait about ten minutes until you feel anything'. Despite gaining no rush, skin-popping was seen to have benefits in avoiding the difficulties in finding and hitting a vein:

I still feel I'm getting somewhere because I actually have given up, you know, digging around for veins and sitting for an hour and a half poking a needle in and out of me with blood dripping, you know, from these holes.

(Male heroin injector)

While the rotation of injection sites to minimize vein deterioration has become a marked feature of harm reduction advice in Britain, many users found themselves with little choice but to inject into hard-to-reach veins or capillaries. One injector, for example, talked about having 'got to the stage where I'd completely ran out of all my veins' having 'been through my wrists, elbows, arms, legs, ankles, neck, everywhere ...'. With particularly 'hard-to-reach' veins, users may ask other users to provide the injection:

I once tried to help a friend find a vein and I remember dotting the syringe all over his chest looking for these loose veins and it was so disgusting, horrible. It's all I can do to inject myself ... I've always found it pretty repulsive.

(Male heroin injector)

One option is the injection of drugs into the vein or capillaries in the groin. Groin injections were seen to carry the most risk or danger of all of the most commonly used injection sites (injection into the penis, for example, being one exception). For some regular injectors, the option of making the transition to groin injections was viewed as a 'risk boundary', as the point at which other (safer) routes of administration were preferred. In fact, most injectors were seen 'to fall just short' of making such a transition because 'they refuse to end up going in the groin'. As commented by one injector:

My arms have been cold and I've been screaming and shouting and trying to get a fix ... The only place I haven't fixed, and I never will do, even if I've used every vein in my body, is my groin.

(Male heroin injector)

For those that did 'end up' injecting into the groin, such action was seen to carry increased risk. Apart from some difficulties in accessing the groin (particularly for women) such that a successful injection is made possible and the associated risks of losing a hit are avoided, the probability of health risks related to injection are increased because of the ease with which 'you go into an artery by accident'. This can mean that there's 'no blood going to all the minor veins' with the consequence of having 'a gangrene leg within sixteen hours'. As explained by one user who saw groin injections as a 'risk boundary':

It's been pointed out to me where the vein is and where the artery is cos they're lying next to each other and so it terrifies me. I've seen people in bad, bad ways . . .

(Male heroin injector)

A groin injector of temazepam described an occasion where her partner, who also injected temazepam into his groin, missed his vein and hit his artery:

Xxxx's gone into his groin and he's missed and he's gone into his artery, and of course, if you do that you feel the heat rush down inside of your leg and it feels like your toes are going to just come right off. It's just so painful, it's absolute agony. A grown man, no matter how strong he is, will cry and cry . . . then, of course, you can lose your leg through that. We've both been lucky and I've got other friends who've been lucky as well, but the luck can't hold out.

(Female heroin injector)

Beyond the increased risks of hitting an artery with the possible consequences of pain or amputation (I've seen people one day without walking sticks and the next day with walking sticks'; 'they took half his hip away'; 'he'd lost both legs and he was in a wheelchair – fucking horrific'), successful groin injections are often associated with increased injection-related damage to the body (and thus also of abscess and infections: 'you get abscesses and it's easier to make a mess of your veins') and with an increased bleeding (and perhaps also of HIV risk). As one injector explained:

Being the groin it can bleed a lot. I mean [her partner] normally stops it but if he's had temazepam he doesn't realise it but he's got blood all over his hand and although I know I won't get any germs from Xxxx . . . I still don't like him walking around touching things. So once he has temazepam I literally have to lead him to the bathroom and make him wash his hands cos I don't want the blood everywhere.

(Female heroin injector)

The most commonly identified risks associated with injecting drug use were those that were perceived to be most immediate. In the context of day to day injecting, interviewees saw the deterioration of injecting sites to introduce a number of health and drug-related risks beyond that of HIV or the transmission of infectious disease. There are clearly a variety of costs and benefits associated with the regular injection of drugs. Dominant epidemiological constructions of risk and danger tend to reduce individual choice and decision making to actions directly associated with HIV risk. This is clearly an inadequate portrayal of the costs and benefits associated with injection as they are described by heroin users themselves.

Risk perception, is clearly *processual.* Individuals' perception of 'risk boundaries' are not context-free or independent of the situations in which interaction takes place. They also change over time. This means that behaviours that once seemed risky may become habitualized and routinized. The act of finding a vein and injecting for many not-yet and non-injectors of heroin might seem to verge towards the bizarre or dangerous. Yet the act of injection, for established injectors, is situated within the realm of the everyday. It is mundane and unspectacular. Preparing for an injection may become something akin to making breakfast or having a drink. Similarly, injecting into groins, once part of daily drug routines may shift, over time, from perceptions which prioritorize cost to perceptions which prioritorize benefit.

The habituation of risk behaviour, where little cost/benefit calculation is made highlights the limitations of conventional risk models that tend to conceptualize risk perception as a function of the severity of the harm and the probability of the risk behaviour occurring (Bloor, 1995). Where risk behaviours become habituated over time (be this injecting, injecting into the groin or unsafe sex) they may be perceived to carry *less* risk, particularly if harm has yet to occur. While dominant models of risk predict that a higher actuality of risk behaviour is accompanied by a higher likelihood of harm (which is apparently why individuals make 'rational choices' to avoid risk), for individuals who actually partake in 'risk behaviours' as part of everyday life, such behaviours may be seen to carry more chance of benefit than cost, particularly over time. In short, whereas predictive models posit that continued risk behaviour becomes *more* risky over time, individuals who actually continue to engage in what were once seen, by themselves or others, as risky behaviours may see such behaviour as increasingly less risky, less unusual, and more mundane.

The ways in which most scientific models predict risk may be at odds with the ways in which risk is perceived. This is largely because they fail to account for how risk perception and behaviour is socially organized. Some behaviours are unlikely to be seen as risky unless they are departures from the norm. I am unlikely to make any sort of 'risk calculation' on what others call 'risk behaviour' if such behaviour to me is simply part and parcel of my everyday life and routine. It is naïve to expect individuals to be making predictive-style 'choices' or 'decisions' on the basis of a cost-benefit analysis every time they partake in what has been defined, by others, as 'risk behaviour'. It is most likely that many people 'decide' to inject heroin in the same way as people drink coffee or smoke tobacco. While individuals may be aware of the risks and costs of these behaviours, such actions probably depend less on calculation than habituation because their functional benefits are inextricably bounded by everyday normal life.

Understanding the context in which injecting occurs, and what injecting actually *means* to those who inject, indicates how HIV risk is perceived in the context of other meanings associated with injecting. The assumptive logic of epidemiological risk models fail to account for how 'choice' is both created and constrained by the everyday realities of social life.

Conclusions

While the word and concept of risk remains key to research on the social aspects of AIDS, there has been a tendency to neglect how risk is actually understood by the participants of research themselves. This chapter has illustrated how social and epidemiological research has played a key role in constructing a limited vision of what risk is and of what risk means to people who use heroin. Social constructions of heroin use and of 'addiction' tend to equate heroin use with injection. Epidemiological constructions of heroin use and risk in the time of AIDS equate injection with infection. Yet, as the data presented in this chapter show, the risks specifically associated with the transmission of infectious disease (be this hepatitis or HIV) are seen as relative concerns by heroin injectors themselves. There are a host of other risks, dangers, costs, benefits and meanings associated with injection that to heroin users may be more important.

In the absence of understanding how HIV-risks are perceived in the context of everyday life, we are left with what appear to be measures without meaning. The obvious and necessary step when researching risk is to understand how risk is perceived among those whom we wish to study. Current scientific definitions of risk among heroin users, which almost exclusively centre on the HIV-risks of injection, may often be at odds with current heroin users' definitions and perceptions of risk. As long as this is the case, interventionists and researchers are left with what can only be described as glimmers of understanding about the social processes which influence how and why heroin users behave as they do.

Acknowledgements

I am particularly grateful for the helpful comments made by Alan Quirk who also undertook fieldwork on this research project. The data presented in this chapter are drawn from Department of Health funded research, which investigated the sexual behaviour and sexual safety of stimulant and opiate users.

Notes

1   See: Jan Zita Grover (1988) 'AIDS: Keywords', in Douglas Crimp (Ed.) *AIDS: Cultural Analysis, Cultural Activism*, Cambridge, MA: MIT Press.
2   This project was funded by the UK Department of Health. Fieldwork was undertaken by Alan Quirk (CRDHB) and Tim Rhodes (CRDHB). See Rhodes, T., Quirk, A.D. and Stimson, G.V. (1995) *Sexual Safety in the Context of Drug Users' Lifestyles: A Qualitative Study Among Users of Opiates and Stimulants*, London: The Centre for Research on Drugs and Health Behaviour (200 Seagrave Road, London, SW6).
3   To 'whack' means to inject, as does 'jack', 'hit', 'bang', 'shoot', 'fix', etc.
4   'Gouching' and to 'gouch' describes the effects commonly associated with having just taken heroin, which are characterized by nodding-off, slowness of speech and lowness of voice. It is sometimes also referred to as being 'on the nod'.
5   'Works' means a needle and syringe.
6   'Chasing' means to smoke heroin by inhaling the fumes once it is heated. The heroin (usually in its 'base' form rather than hydrochloride) once placed on foil is heated from underneath. This practice is known as 'chasing the dragon'. For a description of the mechanics and culture of chasing see Griffiths, P., Gossop, M. and Strang, J. (1994) 'Chasing the dragon: the development of heroin smoking in the United Kingdom', in Strang, J. and Gossop, M. (Eds) *Heroin Addiction and Drug Policy: The British System*, Oxford: Oxford University Press.
7   'Boot' or 'booting' means 'chase' or 'chasing' (see note 6 above). Among London heroin users, it is a phrase used most commonly south of the Thames where 'boot' is a derivative of the rhyming slang 'Boot-Lace, Chase'

References

ADAMS, J. (1995) *Risk*, London: UCL Press.
BANDURA, A. (1977) 'Self-efficacy: towards a unifying theory of behavioural change', *Psychological Review*, **84**, 191–215.
BECK, U. (1992) *Risk Society*, London: Sage.
BECKER, H.M. (1974) The health belief model and personal health behaviour', *Health Education Monographs*, **84**, 191–215.
BERRIDGE, V. (1992) AIDS: history and contemporary history', in HERDT, G. and LINDENBAUM, S. (Eds) *The Time of AIDS: Social Analysis, Theory and Method*, London: Sage.
BLOOR, M. (1995) *The Sociology of HIV Transmission*, London: Sage.
CONNORS, M. (1992) 'Risk perception, risk taking and risk management among intravenous drug users: implications for AIDS prevention', *Social Science and Medicine*, **34**, 591–601.
DOUGLAS, M. (1986) *Risk Acceptability According to the Social Sciences*, London: Routledge and Kegan Paul.
DOUGLAS, M. (1992) *Risk and Blame: Essays in Cultural Theory*, London: Routledge.
FISHBEIN, M. and AZJEN, I. (1975) *Belief, Attitude, Intention and Behaviour; An Introduction*

to Theory and Research, Reading, MA: Addison-Wesley.

FRIEDMAN, S.R., DES JARLAIS, D.C. and WARD, T.P. (1994) 'Social models for changing health-relevant behaviour', in DICLIMENTE, R.J. and PETERSON, J.L. (Eds) *Preventing AIDS: Theories and Methods of Behaviour Interventions*, New York: Plenum.

GIDDENS, A. (1991) *Modernity and Self-Identity in the Late Modern Age*, Cambridge: Polity Press.

KANE, S. (1991) 'HIV, heroin and heterosexual relations', *Social Science and Medicine*, **32**, 1037–991.

KANE, S. and MASON, T. (1992) ' "IV drug users" and "sex partners": the limits of epidemiological categories and the ethnography of risk', in HERDT, G. and LINDENBAUM, S. (Eds) *The Time of AIDS: Social Analysis, Theory and Method*, London: Sage.

PATTON, C. (1990) *Inventing AIDS*, New York: Routledge.

RHODES, T., QUIRK, A. and STIMSON G.V. (1995) *Sexual Safety in the Context of Drug Taking and Sexual Lifestyles*, London: The Centre for Research on Drugs and Health Behaviour.

RHODES, T. and QUIRK, A. (1995) 'Heroin, Risk and Sexual Safety: Some problems for interventions encouraging community change', in RHODES, T. and HARTNOLL, R. (Eds) *AIDS, Drugs and Prevention: Perspectives on Individual and Community Action*, London: Routledge.

RHODES, T., STIMSON, G.V. and QUIRK, A. (forthcoming) 'Sex, drugs, intervention and research: from the individual to the social', *International Journal of the Addictions*.

SCHWARTZ, H. and JACOBS, J. (1979) *Qualitative Sociology: A Method to the Madness*, London: Free Press.

Chapter 10

Sex, Love and Seropositivity: Balancing the Risks

Gill Green

Whilst there is a plethora of studies on the sexual behaviour of 'high-risk' groups, notably men who have sex with men, injecting drug users, sex workers and young people, there are few studies on the sexual behaviour of people with HIV, and a dearth of studies on the emotional impact of HIV on their sexual relationships. Most general texts about 'living with HIV' talk about implications for sexual relationships, and many focus upon the trauma of disclosing one's status to long-term sexual partners (Henderson, 1992; Siegel and Krauss, 1991; Tavanyar, 1992). However, the evidence of emotional disruption is largely restricted to the personal testimonies of people with HIV who talk of the guilt and fears at having sexual relationships, the moral hostility from society, and the loss of sexual confidence that accompanies an HIV seropositive diagnosis (O'Sullivan and Thomson, 1992; Richardson and Bolle, 1992).

This chapter aims to contribute to this skeletal literature by examining how people re-establish interpersonal relationships following an HIV-seropositive diagnosis, and the psychological stress associated with this process. The analysis is set within a discussion of balancing risks in relationships and further develops earlier work on the sexual behaviour of people with HIV and the risk of HIV transmission to seronegative partners (Green, 1994a). In this earlier analysis, three sexual careers among people with HIV were identified. The first is the path of celibacy, which carries no risk of HIV-transmission. The second is that of denial of the possibility of infecting others and failure to modify behaviour. This strategy clearly carries a high risk of infecting sexual partners. The third is the path of behaviour modification and the practice of safer sex (at least most of the time), which enables a sex life to continue and in which the risk of transmission is low. The path an individual chooses may vary with time following diagnosis. Whereas this earlier analysis discussed sex and transmission, the focus here is upon love and relationships, and the two analyses are integrated in the latter section of this paper and developed to build a provisional model of risk-taking in sexual relationships, where one partner knows themselves to be HIV seropositive.

People with HIV who place sexual partners at risk are most often portrayed in the media as 'seeking revenge' by deliberately infecting as many other people as possible. This image has been sufficiently popular and powerful to generate the well-known urban myth in which a person wakes from a one-night stand to find his or her partner gone and 'welcome to the AIDS Club' scrawled in lipstick on the mirror (see Kitzinger, 1993). Research to date has shown that people from all transmission groups, at least occasionally, practise unsafe sex and risk transmitting the virus to seronegative partners (Dublin *et al.*, 1992; Green, 1994a; Hankins *et al.*, 1993; Johnstone *et al.*, 1990; Weatherburn *et al.*, 1993 and White *et al.*, 1993). Exposing others to the virus, however, most often occurs within the context of a loving committed relationship in which sexual partners are fully aware of the risk (Green 1994a; McClean *et al.*, 1994).

It has been suggested that many people disregard the risk of HIV in sexual relationships because loving, or even simply knowing someone can lead people to assume that they are clean and safe (see, for example, Ingham *et al.*, 1991; Weatherburn *et al.*, 1991). The value of personal relationships, affection and trust between partners, often overrides concern about HIV infection (McKeganey and Barnard, 1992). McLean *et al.*, 1994 shows that gay men's perception of the riskiness of unprotected intercourse with their partner is closely related to their emotional involvement with that partner, and that the perceived risk is greatly reduced among those who are 'in love' with their partner compared with those who are not. The maintenance of personal relationships may transcend a concern about HIV, and this would appear to apply to some people who are seropositive.

Risks to sexual health are also taken in order to conceive, as safer sex is incompatible with reproduction. Women seeking semen donors for self-insemination occasionally take risks due to a scarcity of finding a suitable donor (Macaulay *et al.*, 1995). Even given the high risk of HIV transmission, some people in long-term committed relationships are willing to try and conceive with their HIV seropositive partners because they specifically want to have *their* child (Green, 1994b).

Sobo (1993) has identified a number of psycho-social benefits of denial linked to unsafe sex among poor African-American women. Insistence upon safe sex risks verbal or physical abuse, the loss of a partner, and childlessness. Safer sex may also lower self-esteem in that the woman has to acknowledge that her partner may not be faithful to her. Risk denial, fatalistic acceptance and persisting in high-risk behaviour may be a more attractive option. Unsafe sex implies closeness, trust, honesty and commitment and leaves rosy façades and dreams of monogamy and security intact.

From the literature, it is clear that HIV-risk behaviour can only be understood within a holistic context. Each individual has to balance the risk of transmitting HIV against other risks such as the threat to a relationship, or the reproductive limitations, or the loss of self-esteem that may accompany safe sex. This chapter aims to examine the most important factors in the HIV-risk equation.

Methods

A sample of 62 HIV seropositive men and women were asked about the impact that an HIV diagnosis had had upon their sex lives and sexual relationships, as part of an in-depth interview about the psycho-social impact of an HIV diagnosis. The baseline interviews were conducted in 1991–92, follow-up interviews of 40 of the cohort took place a year later, and 33 were re-interviewed in a third 1994 contact. Details of the sample, which was recruited from hospital clinics, voluntary agencies, self-help groups and prisons, are set out in Table 10.1. It included both men and women from all transmission categories; the largest group being those with a history of injecting drug use, reflecting the epidemiology of HIV in Scotland. All respondents were white. Some had been diagnosed several years before the baseline interview and others only a few months beforehand, and most of the

Table 10.1 Details of the sample at time of baseline interview 1991–92

		HIV-seropositive sample	HIV-seronegative sample
Total		62	67
Sex	Men	50	54
	Women	12	13
Transmission category	Gay men	15	14
	Drug users	29	29
	Haemopohilics	10	7
	Other heterosexuals	8	17
No. with AIDS		9	–
Current relationship	Has regular partner	31	33
	No regular partner	31	34
Sexual relationships with other people with HIV	Yes now	8	0
	In the past only	9	9
	Never	36	58
	Missing	9	0

sample were asymptomatic, although some were ill and nine had received a diagnosis of AIDS. In addition, a control group of 67 people who were seronegative was also recruited. The seronegative respondents were broadly matched with the seropositive sample in terms of age, gender and transmission category. They were interviewed once only in 1992.

The diversity of the sample was apparent in their sexual identities, sexual orientations, sexual experience and current relationship status. Among the seropositive sample, there was a vast range in experience, ranging from five who were sexually inexperienced at time of diagnosis to some of the women who had worked as sex workers and reported having had hundreds of sexual partners. Likewise, a few had never had a long-term sexual relationship, whereas others reported more than twenty and half the sample were currently in a long-term relationship at the time of the baseline interview. About one-third of the seropositive sample reported that they had had or were currently in a relationship with someone who was also seropositive.

All the interviews with the seropositive respondents were conducted by myself and a male colleague. Given the huge diversity of experience, this section of the interview schedule was relatively unstructured, consisting of a simple checklist of topic headings, which included whether and how they told sexual partners of their HIV status, their partners' reaction to disclosure, HIV status of partners, emotional impact of HIV on long-term relationships and the impact that this had on life. This approach enabled us to question respondents within their own terms of reference, and the detail, scope and direction of the discussion about sexual relationships was guided largely by cues given by the respondents. One man, for example, was prepared to talk about his sex life but would say nothing about the gender or HIV status of his partner. Some gave long accounts of intimate details of many aspects of their relationships, others talked about their disappointment at and reasons for not having a relationship, and some indicated that they were unwilling or unable to talk at length on this topic. Respondents defined what they considered to be a 'long-term relationship' or 'regular partner', although they were advised that these should normally be relationships that had lasted at least three months. The follow-up interviews asked about changes in sex life that had taken place since the last interview. Questions to the seronegative control group were limited to number of regular and casual partners, frequency of condom use and HIV status of current and previous partners.

Emotional Impact of HIV upon Sexual Relationships

HIV-seropositive respondents were as likely as the seronegative controls to be in a committed sexual relationship. At time of diagnosis and at each interview, about half the seropositive sample reported being in a long-term relationship.

Table 10.2 Emotional impact of HIV upon sexual relationships and psychological stress

Impact	N*	Psychological stress
Restricted access: ineligible as long-term partner; lack of confidence	22	High
Extra strain: difficulties about disclosure; sexual problems; family formation; illness; disequilibrium; guilt	36	Medium
Closer: partner's acceptance; sharing illness; met after both had been diagnosed positive	16	Low
No change: HIV not an integral part of relationship	18	Low

*Number of respondents who have reported this in any relationship

Between the first and last interview (about three years later) over one-third of respondents reported a change in relationship status or partner. It would therefore appear that HIV status does not greatly alter the likelihood of being in a relationship, but the qualitative data collected from the seropositive respondents suggest that they perceive HIV to have a major impact upon relationships. Table 10.2 identifies the four principal themes that emerged from the data. These are restricted access, extra strain, special closeness, and the lack of impact that HIV has upon relationships. Each of these is discussed below. The numbers of respondents who mentioned these aspects in any relationship they have had since diagnosis is indicated on Table 10.2. A broad assessment of the psychological stress associated with each theme is also indicated. This assessment is based on careful analysis of the content and tone of the interviews with the seropositive respondents.

Restricted access

Twenty-two respondents felt that being HIV-seropositive restricted their access to long-term relationships. Many reported that they felt ineligible as a long-term partner as, having a limited life span, they would be unable to settle down and plan a long-term future. Nor would they be able to have a family as this would risk transmitting the virus to their partner and any potential child. This is well-illustrated by the following quotation from a male injecting drug-user in his early twenties who was talking about why he had ended a relationship with a woman he described as the 'love of his life':

R12:   She wanted to keep the relationship going but I just wanted it to end.

GG: Why was that?

R12:   It could not go anywhere, the relationship. You could have safe sex but at the end of the day it is whether you can carry on and settle down and get married and have children. That is what you want in life. Not to have safe sex all the time.

The psychological cost associated with feelings of ineligibility was extremely high. Not only did these respondents feel debarred from having fulfilling committed sexual relationships, but they were also denied a much-desired future and had to reformulate their expected life trajectories in the light of HIV.

Access to relationships was also restricted due to lack of confidence and a belief that no one would want a relationship with anybody who was HIV seropositive. This lack of confidence prevented relationships forming, as in the case of a person with haemophilia who said he had always felt awkward about starting relationships and that since his diagnosis: 'I mean even thinking about taking up with a girl, you know. I just don't know how the hell to approach it.' Even the more sexually assured prior to diagnosis reported that their sexual confidence waned following diagnosis as HIV made them, in their eyes, a less desirable partner. According to a charismatic gay man in his thirties:

R24   It's more difficult, there is no doubt about it, I mean I forget what it's like to be negative. But I think for people who don't know their status, the announcement somewhere on the line, you know, that I've got HIV is not maybe a great turn on, and even in a relationship ... there is the concern that what if you become sick. I think that's a legitimate area. There's no answer to it but it does colour any kind of relationship.

In the main, those who reported that HIV restricted their access to relation-ships were the least sexually experienced, had least sexual confidence prior to diagnosis and felt highly stigmatized by HIV. Many of the people with haemophilia, for example, had been diagnosed when they were adolescents, others reported a past history of difficulty with relationships due to the stigma associated with haemophilia, and, unlike injecting drug users or gay men were more socially isolated from other people affected by HIV and thus more stigmatized by it. High levels of stigma and isolation were also reported by those infected heterosexually, many of whom felt debarred from forming relationships following diagnosis.

Extra strain

Fifty two respondents had had a sexual relationship since diagnosis, and 36 of them felt that HIV had had a detrimental effect, particularly those in discordant couples. Disclosing one's HIV status to partners caused enormous stress, especially if this also entailed disclosure of a history of drug use too. Two people mentioned that they had felt suicidal before doing so fearing rejection, others said that they had only been able to disclose when drunk and then did so insensitively, and some were unable to disclose at all. Almost one-third had been rejected by their partners and occasionally this was accompanied by verbal abuse or physical violence. One woman said her husband had poured bleach over her, another had been called a 'slag', and at least three respondents had been accused of infidelity. Sometimes partners would initially react well and then gradually reject their partner, as in the case of the female injecting drug user quoted below who told her new partner about her drug use shortly after meeting him and about her HIV status a week later:

> R34: Well when the relationship first started I told him about myself and things and I thought he was really understandable, but then after a month or so he changed, he just – it was like he was still coming to see me and things but he started to like – och he just stopped like, we stopped having sex. He used to make excuses, and then eventually it got to the stage where he was even scared to kiss me . . . It was a right let down, you know. It took me months to get over it. . . . It'll take me a long time to trust a man again.

Extra strain and stress upon relationships were also reported by those who had successfully negotiated disclosure. Sexual problems with their partner following diagnosis was frequently reported. This was related to the fear of transmission, and often had severe repercussions upon the emotional relationship. Some said that their partners had 'gone off sex' as they were worried about being infected. More commonly, it was the respondents who were concerned about transmitting HIV to their partner. Three people whose relationships had continued following their diagnosis, for example, had decided to stop having sex with their partner. Others continued to have sex but reported enjoying it much less.

Family formation was another source of tension between couples. Many couples desired children, and about one-third of the heterosexual respondents had tried to conceive a child since their diagnosis (Green, 1994b). This topic was sometimes a source of tension between couples particularly in discordant couples where the man was seropositive. Several male respondents reported that their partner wanted to have *their* child, and that they felt uncomfortable given the risk of transmission that this entailed.

Illness and impending death also put relationships under strain. Whilst it occasionally brought couples closer together, it could also drive them apart. Respondents reported that some partners were unable to relax about their health. As one respondent said: 'she starts greeting (crying) every time I say I don't feel well', and another man said that when he had gone into hospital with shingles, his partner looked as if 'that was me and I was coming out in a pine box'.

Perhaps the principal source of strain was the imbalanced relationships that tended to emerge among discordant couples. This disequilibrium could lead to over-dependency or over-commitment and was often a source of tension. It is well illustrated by the following quotation from a young man with haemophilia who had recently come through a harrowing end to a relationship:

> R14: If someone decides knowing I am HIV positive to sleep with me I feel they are making a major commitment that normally you would not do if you were sleeping with somebody. They are taking extra commitment. It is easier for me because there is no risk for me ... That is why Jane and I lasted so long in the end ... There was a lot of emotional blackmail which was HIV related and which maintained the relationship for a year longer than it would normally have gone on. It made it a lot more extreme and a lot more intense, and a lot more problematic. Just crazy basically, it got to crazy levels which would never have happened if it had not been for HIV.

Related to this disequilibrium is the guilt felt by many respondents in their relationships. Respondents expressed guilt about being ill or being dependent on their partner, and, all those with HIV-seronegative partners, felt guilty about potentially infecting them.

In general, those who reported that HIV put extra strain upon their relationships had been in a relationship when they were diagnosed. They had thus experienced a relationship which was relatively unaffected by HIV and it would often flounder following diagnosis due to the extra strains that HIV imposed upon it. HIV was also blamed for destroying or creating problems in relationships that had been formed since diagnosis. Several respondents, however, were clear that deterioration of a relationship was not caused by HIV.

Special closeness

Sixteen respondents said that HIV had fostered closeness between them and their partner. This included almost all of those who had recently disclosed to their partner and were enjoying a 'honeymoon period' following their partner's acceptance, as illustrated by a male prisoner whose girlfriend had recently found out about his HIV status:

R7: She said it changes nothing you know and the relationship continued. You didnae know what that made me feel like back on the clouds again. I really thought that everything would have finished there and then ... As I say she is not the strongest of people but she has proved to me how strong she must be. The welfare has been on her back, her mum's been on her back. She has decided herself you know. For the first time in my life someone has made me feel really wanted.

A closer relationship was also reported by respondents after the onset of illness when they realised the full extent of their partner's concern and commitment. Also, most of the couples who had met after both had been diagnosed seropositive reported that they had atypically close relationships, at least in the short term. Their relief at having found a partner who was going through the same experience, and the lack of complications often faced by discordant couples, fostered an open and honest relationship:

GG: How has HIV affected your relationship?
R6: I think it is better because I am not prepared to put up with second best anymore. If things don't come up to my expecta- tions I just get shot of them ... I think Eric (her HIV-positive partner) feels that way too. Just not got time for shit anymore ... It is funny I have just never felt about anybody before the way I feel about him.
GG: Why do you think that is?
R6: Probably because the kind of relationship I want now, as I say I want quality instead of quantity you know. I let him see me warts and all ... With Eric it's if you don't like me that is the way I am you know.

Gay men were proportionally more likely to report closer relationships than other respondents. As they and their sexual partners belong to a 'risk group', they were more likely to find a seropositive partner, or to meet with a sympathetic response from a partner when they disclosed their HIV status.

No change

Eighteen respondents said that they had experienced relationships in which their HIV status had had minimal or no impact. Despite rigorous probing in the interview, they insisted that 'it has not made any difference', 'we don't dwell on it', 'we fight and argue like any other couple' and 'we just try to live normal lives and do the things that normal couples do'. They preferred to put HIV to one side and forget about it as much as possible, often with their partners' collusion.

Those who reported that HIV was not an integral part of their emotional relationships often chose to downplay or ignore the implications of HIV in their sexual relationship, and sometimes had unsafe sex. They included those who found condoms impeded emotional closeness, people who had a seropositive partner, and three people who had not told their partner of their HIV status. They were all asymptomatic and were dealing with HIV by giving it little significance in the functioning of their everyday lives.

The psychological stress associated with the 'no change' strategy was low, at least in the short term, as HIV could be temporarily 'put to one side' and the relationship could flourish. It could, however, have very serious repercussions in the long term among those who chose to downplay or ignore HIV in their sexual behaviour. Some of those having unsafe sex with negative partners were concerned about infecting their partners, and one man who had infected his partner, witnessed her death from AIDS. The guilt of those who had infected their partners, and/or the anger directed at them from their partners, normally made it impossible to sustain the relationship:

R12: It made me feel a bit guilty but it's hard to deliberately point the finger at me when she had slept with other people and she was more or less clutching at straws. OK it could have been me that infected her but she never knew that for certain.

GG: So what was it that finally split you up?

R12: Just her more or less constantly tormenting me saying I had infected her which she didn't know for sure ... I just couldn't handle it.

Most who reported 'no change' and failed to modify their sexual behaviour were drug users; the day-to-day benefits of this strategy of denial was not out of keeping with their relatively chaotic lifestyles.

Sexual Careers

It was noted in an earlier analysis (Green, 1994a) that the sexual path an individual takes is flexible and may vary over time following diagnosis. Many initially opt for celibacy or denial but may later feel sufficiently sexually confident to adopt the third path of behaviour modification and safer sex. And those who initially respond by practising safer sex may change in response to changing circumstances, such as meeting a new partner with whom they want to have a child.

The typology of the emotional impact upon relationships outlined above is also flexible and no one person nor any one relationship is necessarily confined to any one category. Seven people, for example, who in the first interview felt ineligible as a long-term partner had formed relationships a year or two years later. One began an intense and very committed relationship with someone with another chronic illness, two formed relationships with people who worked in the HIV field, another had met a seropositive partner, and three had negotiated relationships in which sex was exclusively non-penetrative. Likewise some relationships which were initially closer because of HIV or unchanged by it, had collapsed by the time of the follow-up interviews. This was usually in response to HIV-related factors such as death of a partner, the onset of illness whereby denial became a less-appropriate strategy, or the seroconversion of a partner, but sometimes to factors unrelated to HIV such as imprisonment or emigration. And some of those who reported that HIV put enormous strain upon their relationships had decided to stop seeking a long-term partner.

It is difficult, however, to discern a 'career' in emotional relationships following diagnosis. Whilst it is tempting to assume that individuals progress from feeling they can never have a relationship with anybody to having one which is stressful to having one which is closer or unaffected by HIV, this was rarely noted to be the case. Personality, lifestyle or sexual identity of the individual and the *modus operandi* generated by each relationship were the factors that were more likely to mediate the impact of HIV upon relationships than time since diagnosis.

Emotional Impact, Sexual Path and Risk

Combining the results of the earlier analysis about sexual behaviour with the current analysis of the emotional impact upon relationships, suggests that both are, to some extent, interrelated (see Table 10.3). While it should be reiterated that all the categories are flexible, and that the match between sexual path and emotional impact is not a perfect fit, it is nevertheless possible to identify a degree of overlap, and this gives some insight into why some people with HIV may put sexual partners at high risk of transmission.

Restricted access to relationships is an inevitable consequence of the sexual path of celibacy for all except the three respondents who were in committed relationships when diagnosed and responded to it by stopping sexual relations with their partner whilst continuing the relationship. Whilst this path carries no risk of transmission, the psychological stress associated with it is high. All those who felt that their access to relationships was restricted

Table 10.3 Emotional impact, sexual path and transmission and psychological risk associated with it

Impact	Sexual path	Transmission risk	Psychological stress
Restricted access	celibacy	nil	high
Extra strain	behav mod	low	medium
Closer	behav mod	low	low
No change	a) behav mod	low	low
	b) denial	high	low

expressed a desire to have a regular committed partnership, except for one single woman who reported that being on her own had been a rewarding experience and was now her preferred option. For the others, however, restricted access to relationships was a source of loneliness and discontent.

Respondents who believed HIV put extra strain on their relationship tended to practise some form of behaviour modification. In general they would practise safer sex with occasional lapses in order to conceive, or at moments of intense emotion. Whilst the transmission risk associated with this path is relatively low, the psychological stress is relatively high as HIV has a detrimental effect upon the emotional relationship, which for many is the central pivot of their lives.

With four exceptions, those experiencing closer relationships practised safer sex even if their partner was also seropositive, in order to minimize the risk of cross-infection. Of the exceptions, two stopped having sex with their partners; one of whom sought sex from casual partners (as did his partner) and the other reported that sex between him and his wife had never been an important part of their relationship. The two other exceptions were both injecting drug users, one of whom had a seropositive partner and felt the risk of cross-infection was a small risk to pay for the closeness that spontaneous sex promoted between them, and the other gradually stopped using condoms as the relationship between him and his partner became more established. Overall, for those in this category the risk of transmission is low and, as long as the relationship continues to be close, the psychological stress is also relatively low.

Those who reported no change in their emotional relationships followed two distinct sexual paths. First, there were those who modified their sexual behaviour and practised safer sex with their partner, even though they chose to downplay or ignore HIV in other aspects of the relationship. The other slightly larger group were those who followed the path of denial about infecting a sexual partner. All but one of the 'deniers' were injecting drug users (the one exception was a heterosexual man who was ill-informed about the risk of sexual transmission to partners). In this scenario the risk of transmission to partners is extremely high, but the psychological stress, at least in the short term, is relatively low. In the longer-term, however, the psychological cost may be extremely high for those who infect their partners.

One can thus see the psychological benefits of high-risk sexual behaviour within regular relationships at least in the short term, and the psychological cost of the nil transmission risk option. The path of celibacy that puts other people at least risk and elicits minimum public opprobrium may cause much personal unhappiness, whereas denial which puts others at high risk and is associated with maximum public opprobrium may cause least disruption in the short term. In short, the possibility of infecting a partner or being subject to public disapproval (or even imprisonment in some parts of the world) may be a price worth paying for the short-term benefits of a 'carefree' emotional and sexual relationship. In many cases, the partner may collude with or even instigate this assessment and, balancing the relative risks, decide that the maintenance of the relationship transcends the risk of HIV-transmission.

Such findings confirm the primacy of personal relationships in risk-taking, at least for some people with HIV and their partners. It gives us some insight into how people with HIV balance the sexual risk equation. Other factors that make-up the equation are the social and psychological risks of being single and having no relationship, renouncing family formation and intentions to have children, losing one's partner, and relinquishing denial as a coping strategy.

Taking risks within relationships is part of a long cultural tradition in a society in which we are all potentially 'fools for love'. Risk-taking is a common feature of sexual relationships: the risk of being emotionally or economically dependent, the risk of falling pregnant or contracting an STD, the risk of domestic violence, etc. The risk of HIV-transmission occurs within this cultural context; and has to be balanced against other risks within relationships or the risk of not having a relationship at all.

Acknowledgements

This research was carried out at the MRC Medical Sociology Unit, Glasgow University and funded by the Medical Research Council of Great Britain. Thanks are due to Steve Platt who played a major role in the overall design of the study and conducted half of the baseline interviews. I am also extremely grateful to the respondents who were prepared to discuss intimate, and highly stigmatizing, areas of their lives, and to Steve Green, Miriam Guthrie, Harry Meany, Helen Mien and Anne Pinkman for their assistance with recruitment. Thanks also to colleagues Graham Hart, Rory Williams and Danny Wight for their helpful comments on an earlier draft.

References

DUBLIN, S., ROSENBERG, P.S. and GOEDERT, J.J. (1992) 'Patterns and predictors of high-risk sexual behavior in female partners of HIV-infected men with hemophilia', *AIDS*, **6**, 475–82.

GREEN, G. (1994a) 'Positive sex: the sexual relationships of a cohort of men and women following an HIV-positive diagnosis', in AGGLETON, P., DAVIES, P. and HART, G. (Eds) *AIDS: Foundations for the Future*, London: Taylor & Francis.

GREEN, G. (1994b) 'The reproductive careers of a cohort of men and women following an 'HIV-positive diagnosis', *Journal of Biosocial Science*, **26**, 409–15.

HANKINS, C., GENDRON,S., LAMPING, D., LAPOINTE, N., KIELO, J. and GAUTHIER, S. (1993) 'Does an HIV-positive test result improve a woman's sex life?', poster (PO-D20-3974) 'presented at IXth International Conference on AIDS, Berlin.

HENDERSON, S. (1992) 'Living with the virus: perspectives from HIV-positive women in London', in DORN, N., HENDERSON, S. and SOUTH, N. (Eds) *AIDS: Women, Drugs and Social Care*, London: Taylor & Francis.

INGHAM, R., WOODCOCK, A. and STENNER, K. (1991) 'Getting to know you ... young people's knowledge of their partners at first intercourse', *Journal of Community and Applied Psychology*, **1**(2), 117–32.

JOHNSTONE, F., MACCALLUM, L. and RIDDELL, R. (1990) 'Contraceptive use in HIV infected women', *British Journal of Family Planning*, **16**, 106–8.

KITZINGER, J. (1993) 'Understanding AIDS: Researching audience perceptions of Acquired Immune Deficiency Syndrome', in ELDRIDGE, J. (Ed.) *Getting the Message*, London: Routledge.

MACAULAY, L., KITZINGER, J., GREEN, G. and WIGHT, D. (1995) 'Risks, relationships and reproduction: the impact of HIV on women seeking to conceive outside a steady heterosexual relationship', *AIDS Care* 7, 3, 261–76.

MCKEGANEY, N. and BARNARD, M. (1992) *AIDS, Drugs and Sexual Risk: Lives in the Balance*, Milton Keynes: Open University Press.

MCLEAN, J., BOULTON, M., BROOKES, M., LAKHANI, D., FITZPATRICK, R., DAWSON, J., MCKECHNIE, R. and HART, G. (1994) 'Regular partners and risky behaviour: why do gay men have unprotected intercourse?' *AIDS Care*, **9**(3), 331–41.

O'SULLIVAN, S. and THOMSON, K. (Eds) (1992) *Positively Women: Living with AIDS*, London: Sheba.

RICHARDSON, A. and BOLLE, D. (Eds) (1992) *Wise Before Their Time: people with AIDS and HIV talk about their lives*, London: Harper Collins.

SIEGEL, K. and KRAUSS, B.J. (1991) 'Living with HIV infection: adaptive tasks of seropositive gay men', *Journal of Health and Social Behavior*, **32**, 17–32.

SOBO, E.J. (1993) 'Inner-city women and AIDS: the psycho-social benefits of unsafe sex', *Culture, Medicine and Psychiatry*, **17**, 455–485.

TAVANYAR, J. (1992) *The Terrence Higgins Trust HIV/AIDS Book*, London: Thorsons.

WEATHERBURN, P., HUNT, A.J., DAVIES, P.M., COXON, A.P.M. and McMANUS, T.J. (1991) 'Condom use in a large cohort of homosexually active men in England and Wales', *AIDS Care*, **3**(1), 31–41.

WEATHERBURN, P., DAVIES, P.M., HICKSON, F.C.I., COXON, A.P.M. and McMANUS, T.J. (1993) 'Sexual behaviour among HIV antibody positive gay men', poster (PO-D20-

3996) presented at IXth International Conference on AIDS, Berlin.

WHITE, D., PHILLIPS, K., MULLEADY, G. and CUPITT, C. (1993) 'Sexual issues and condom use among injecting drug users', *AIDS Care* 5(4), 381–91.

Chapter 11

One of Us, One of Them, or One of Those? The Construction of Identity and Sexuality in Relation to HIV/AIDS

Philip Gatter

It is commonly said that HIV and AIDS have forced a complex re-examination of sexuality and its relationship to identity. At the individual level, they direct attention to our sexual behaviours (Bayer, 1989; Davies and Project SIGMA, 1992; Earickson, 1990; Pollak *et al.*, 1992: 85–102). Collectively, through their symbolic and political weight, they force us to re-examine who we are, as a matter of survival (Crimp, 1988; Kayal, 1993; Watney, 1993). Third, and perhaps most crucially, questions of communitarian values are raised: individual behaviours and collective identities may be logically distinct, yet in the real world, and if we are to overcome AIDS, they must be inseparable (Holleran, 1987; Kayal, 1986). In Britain this is most obviously the case for gay men and gay communities.

This chapter focuses on the relationship of sexual identity to HIV/AIDS from an anthropological perspective. The title draws attention to the fact that identity, and its attribution, is a matter of perspective, and has to be understood at a collective as well as individual level. Only one academic perspective is offered here: one which has perhaps been less well developed than others, and one which may be controversial for a gay author writing of gay community, since it argues that identities become vehicles for legitimacy claims, claims which are articulated as resource demands on AIDS Service Organizations.

In terms of academic debate, much has been made in psychology, and to a lesser degree in social psychology and sociology, of how HIV/AIDS influences self-perception, especially via social attitudes and media representations (Altman, 1986; Beeson *et al.*, 1986; Weitz, 1989). This is counterbalanced by more social analyses, for example of HIV/AIDS volunteerism, as a possible manifestation of a New Social Movement with the possibility of new identities forming within and around it (Gamson, 1989). These academic contributions do not exist in a vacuum: researchers are drawn to the work by altruistic as well as selfish motives, and much of the funding is made available on the grounds that research might make a difference to individuals and groups outside the academy. The obverse of this is that individuals and organizations working for HIV prevention and care link into social science research, to make use of it, and to criticize it.

> ... the sciences of epidemiology and behavioural and social science research can be harnessed as powerful allies, rather than enemies, of community responses to AIDS. In describing evidence from the medical and social sciences literature, I have sought to demonstrate how those disciplines can help ordinary gay men concerned about HIV to explain the importance of grass-roots activities and argue for work targeting gay men to be given its due priority.
>
> (King, 1993: xii–xiii)

This quotation informs the perspective that will be adopted here: identity is an arena for *contest* among and between those who contemplate and those who act (and those doing both) in relation to HIV/AIDS. It is informative to view identity as a cultural product, a particular discourse emerging in specific historical and political circumstances (see Weeks, 1986). Further, it is important to recognize that identity is never just about itself. In the case of AIDS activism it becomes a vehicle for developing legitimate claims on scarce resources (health education, care services, etc) through asserting and demonstrating the legitimacy of such claims.

In reference to gay men and communities in Britain, the question becomes: 'who do we mean by gay men; who is the "we" doing the talking, and to what ends?' The answers are not obvious. In the quotation above, qualifying gay men as 'ordinary' apparently brushes away any need to problematize; yet the effect is only transitory. The primary aim of this chapter is to apply a critical discourse perspective to a number of voices that argue about and for gay men in relation to HIV/AIDS in Britain and elsewhere in the west.

Questioning Identity: Gay Men and AIDS

The significance of gay sexual identity for HIV transmission has been extensively explored in relation to individual sexual behaviour, particularly the lack of fit between identity and behaviour (Altman, 1986; Dowsett *et al.*, 1992; Davies, 1987, Davies *et al.*, 1992; Fitzpatrick, *et al.*, 1989; Kippax *et al.*,

1992; Watney, 1993; Weatherburn *et al.*, 1990; Weeks, 1986). The focus in this chapter will instead be accounts of gay men as collectivities or communities, beginning with social science accounts and then moving to activist statements, though, as argued above, the two are often linked either overtly or implicitly.

Many of the sociological contributions in this area have considered sexual identity as manifest in self-consciously gay HIV/AIDS organizations. Writers have drawn attention to a need to understand more fully the wider dynamics of gay community, in relation, for example, to individual knowledge and decisions about HIV- risk behaviour (Bolton, 1992; Parker, 1992). Activists such as Edward King argue that the informal role of gay community has been critical in limiting the extent of the HIV epidemic in Britain (King, 1993); yet very little empirical research exists exploring precisely how membership of community influences HIV outcomes for individuals. The matter is dealt with, though not entirely satisfactorily, by Kippax *et al.* in their work on Australia (1992, 1993).

For historical reasons, the first substantive analyses of gay HIV/AIDS organizations have arisen in the United States of America. Organizations such as Gay Men Fighting AIDS (GMFA) in Britain are comparatively young, and although the Terrence Higgins Trust has been responding to AIDS since 1982, and London Gay Switchboard (now London Lesbian and Gay Switchboard) from the same time, there is no major sociological (as opposed to historical) study of their role and activities (Berridge and Strong, 1992). Examples of such analyses from the States are numerous by comparison (Appleby and Sosnowitz, 1987; Arno, 1986; Katoff and Dunne 1988; Kobasa, 1990). Two accounts are of particular interest in the perspectives they offer and the different kinds of organization they analyse: ACTUP (AIDS Coalition to Unleash Power) and GMHC (Gay Men's Health Crisis).

Gays and Thespians: ACTUP San Francisco

Josh Gamson's sophisticated analysis of ACTUP San Francisco attempts to theorize the organization as arguably an example of a New Social Movement (Eder, 1985; Habermas, 1981; Offe, 1985; Touraine, 1985). Unlike social movements founded in the 1960s, which focused on social divisions such as class and gender, and were strongly influenced by Marxist thinking and politics, ACTUP is a movement organized around identity linked to lifestyle; specifically gay male urban identity. The broad aims of ACTUP, for Gamson, are social justice, by which he means ensuring broader access to HIV treatments and safer sex education; ensuring that those who do research into HIV/AIDS should be accountable to affected people; and ensuring that changes should be made to the distribution of decision-making power and resources in favour of these people. To achieve these aims, ACTUP organizes activities that, often in an expressive and theatrical manner, call attention to the connections between cultural definitions and responses to AIDS, while also attacking its hegemonic representations.

From participant observation in ACTUP, Gamson inferred three apparent confusions within the organization: a lack of a clear definition of the audience for whom expressive actions are intended, coupled to a loose organizational structure rendering focused planning and action difficult; an explicit aim to be an inclusive organization, whilst the majority membership continues to be white middle class gay men in their 20s and 30s; and an apparent tension within the organization between gay politics and AIDS politics. Gamson concluded that these confusions were related to a central issue: who was the 'enemy' ACTUP was trying to fight? At different times, different kinds of foe were apparent: clearly visible controllers of resources, such as the state and corporations; the invisible, abstract, disembodied, ubiquitous process of normalization, i.e. the normalization through labelling in which everyone except one's own 'community' of the denormalized (and its supporters) is involved; and an intermediate enemy: those institutions that act as the channels through which normalization operates (chiefly the media and medical science).

The major theoretical claim of Gamson's study is that the presence and effects of normalization show that ACTUP is responding to a gradual historical shift toward a form of domination in which power is maintained through a normalizing process, rather than identifiable persons and repressive institutions (Foucault, 1977). While domination is increasingly abstracted and invisible, the dominated become embodied and visible (marked by stigmatization), and increasingly the focus of attention. People effectively come to dominate themselves through being confronted with the threat of being devalued as abnormal.

> When power is effected through categorisation, identity is often built on the very categories it resists. ACTUP's expressive actions, in this light, are part of a continuing process of actively forging a gay identity while challenging the process through which it is formed *for* gay people ... identity-oriented actions accept the labels, and symbolic actions disrupt and resignify them.
>
> (Gamson, 1989: 44)

Since this enemy is invisible and disembodied, it can only really be tackled through the manipulation of symbols.

Why then is it a problem for ACTUP to include other than white middle-class gay men? Gamson argues that the process of label disruption is most accessible to the white middle classes since they draw on knowledge of mainstream culture as privileged members, regardless of sexual orientation;

they can, therefore, disrupt the norms of the mainstream by drawing on familiar vocabulary, whereas more marginal groups, such as ethnic minorities, cannot do so with such ease. But why also does the shifting constituency remain gay? Gamson argues that the process of normalization is one of ACTUP's main enemies:

> AIDS is a gay disease because AIDS has been made to attribute viral disease to sexual deviance. Separating AIDS politics from gay politics would be to give up the fight against normalisation. Yet joining the two politics poses the risk of losing the fight in that it confirms the very connection it attempts to dispel.
>
> (Gamson, 1989: 52)

On the one hand, then, ACTUP is driven toward inclusiveness because other populations are increasingly affected by HIV and are in a similar fight for material resources. Yet resisting the label GAY=AIDS means first accepting it, then redefining and thus reappropriating it, situating ACTUP in the wider label disruption process of queer politics (see Outrage mock funerals, or canonizations by the Order of Perpetual Indulgence). This drives ACTUP away from inclusiveness.

Gamson's analysis is significant for several reasons. First, it draws attention to a collective, intersubjective level of gay identity in relation to HIV/AIDS, one which can be invoked, and modified, through cultural symbols: it is not monolithic. Second, it becomes clear that sexuality is not a priori segregated from other aspects of identity in analysing collective identity. ACTUP's dynamics have to be understood as expressing class and race dimensions as well. Yet at the same time, it becomes clear that at the level of meaning HIV/AIDS is a different phenomenon for gay men than for women or members of minority ethnic groups, because of a wider set of cultural associations between AIDS, disease, death, deviance, and gay sexuality.

Finally, Gamson illustrates how the social and cultural manifestation of AIDS militates against gay organizations forming wider alliances. His analysis lends weight to those activists who argue for a regaying of AIDS (e.g. King, 1993; Scott, 1992; Watney, 1993), though perhaps for different reasons. On grounds of logic and organizational harmony, his evidence could be used to support an argument for the targeting of resources to specific groups at risk of HIV; an argument made more in terms of morality, ethics and politics by activists. This is perhaps a key difference between social scientists' insights into AIDS-related organizations and the concerns of gay activists, even though both groups may reach the same conclusions in terms of recommendations for policy.

GMHC and AIDS Volunteerism

Philip Kayal's study of GMHC concerns the nature of gay AIDS volunteerism and its relation to gay community. Based on participant observation and interviews conducted during several years as a volunteer it is a thorough examination of the nature of gay men's volunteering in relation to AIDS and to the wider American culture of volunteerism (see Arno, 1986, 1988; Babchuk *et al.*, 1960; Chambers, 1985; Chambre, 1991). Sociologically, Kayal focuses on the relation between subjectivity and community as necessary to an understanding of volunteerism. He argues that certain structural features of AIDS forced gay men to action; features that were not present for other members of society:

> Unfortunately, class and life-style variations, personal and political ideologies, education and other factors all fragment female and minority populations, making their interests less compatible or uniform. Yet the way HIV spreads and who it touches brings all gays together into one interest group automatically and immediately.
>
> (Kayal, 1993: 111–2)

Kayal reasons that AIDS literally attacks the fabric of gay community (life-threatening illness mediated sexually); this is not so for heterosexuals. But this is not sufficient to explain who volunteers and why. In his typology of GMHC volunteers, Kayal goes on to show that gay volunteers typically are out of the closet, accepting of their own and others' sexuality, and politically gay (Kayal, 1993: 120). They are also relatively high achievers, both educationally and occupationally (Kayal, 1993: 122). This tension between laying claim to AIDS as a 'pan-gay' phenomenon yet finding a differentiated response is also present in activist calls for regaying AIDS, a point taken up below.

Kayal's most illuminating thesis concerns the way in which AIDS has informed gay identity through demanding participation in, and transformation of, community. Remarkably, gay men of high social status have turned altruistically to support others with whom they are connected only by being gay, and perform for them menial and sometimes physically unpleasant tasks ('dirty work'); caring acts deemed culturally the province of women (and therefore not highly valued). Rooted in a history of gay activism, the gay response to AIDS, therefore, can be seen both as a reaction to institutionalized homophobia (Kayal, 1993: 29) and a journey toward overcoming internalized homophobia (Kayal, 1993: 96). Gay men, whether HIV positive or not, volunteer for PWAs (Persons with AIDS) because they are all members of a 'community for rejected others seen as the extended self' (Kayal, 1993: 110).

The master concept here for Kayal is 'bearing witness', a concept having explicit theological origins. Originally it referred to Christ's bearing of others' sins.

... bearing witness is the willingness to take on the sufferings of others as if it were one's own, but in a way that brings carepartners into deep conversation with themselves about their own value or sacredness as human beings.

(Kayal, 1993: 14)

Crucially, bearing witness means that AIDS volunteerism empowers the gay community through connecting individual and collective interests (Kayal, 1993: 8). At times the tone is evangelical: bearing witness puts us in touch with our sacred selves and a lower case god. But the transformative power of community participation leads Kayal to conclusions regarding the wider question of what community means, and the practical issue of containing HIV.

Community is significant for individual behaviour since it influences mental, physical, and spiritual health. Whereas psychologists might look on sexual risk behaviour as an individual aberration, they ignore the sociological insight that social structure and self-esteem, belonging and estrangement, shape the context in which sexual behaviours occur. For Kayal, AIDS is, ironically, healing for gay men and gay community, since it challenges an earlier 'sexcentricity' of gay life (Kayal, 1993: 94) and forces a greater sense of collective responsibility, independent of erotic desire. Through demanding nurturing and caring, it also questions a masculinist, patriarchal gay sexuality which merely reflects and reproduces a sexist heterosexual order. Further development of this kind of community may be important for containing HIV, for two reasons. Raised self-esteem encourages gay men to take greater responsibility for themselves and others, whereas gayness purely as sexual self-gratification does not. Second, self-acceptance through growth in community makes resort to anonymous, instrumental, alienated sexual connection unnecessary: Kayal sees this as a risk for HIV transmission (Kayal, 1993: 95)

In effect, safer-sex proponents operate conservatively rather than inventively in the approach, goals, and techniques they propose, such as eroticizing condom use. By devising solutions that promote safer sexual practices but that leave instrumental relations untouched, gay sexual activity will remain shaped by the heterosexist order.

(Kayal, 1993: 94)

The problem with Kayal's analysis is that it tends to conflate his empirical findings with an unacknowledged moral position. Whilst not sex-negative, he does come across as 'touchy feely' in an implicitly Christian manner. In contrast, Edward King, as an activist writer in Britain, draws on the empirical work of SIGMA Research (formerly Project SIGMA) to argue that discussion of anonymous, instrumental sex is a red herring in relation to considerations of HIV risk since unprotected anal sex (the only sexual activity for gay men bearing a significant risk for HIV transmission) is rare outside of sustained intimate relationships. The sense of community which Kayal discusses may have value for gay men, but the connection with HIV prevention is not established. Many gay activists in Britain and the United States of America, in unison with many sex researchers, would strongly disagree with Kayal's conclusions cited in the quotation above.

Community and Identity: Activist Perspectives.

Both Gamson and Kayal have produced academic analyses of community and identity in relation to gay men and AIDS. Yet this does not deny a personal as well as a professional involvement with the issues: Kayal self-consciously writes as a gay sociologist, and his emphasis on the spiritual dimension of gay community is clearly personal. It is instructive to turn now to statements from activist commentators, particularly those working for the regaying of AIDS, to further a discourse perspective on identity and AIDS. Again I have chosen a particular text to examine: in this case *Safety in Numbers* by Edward King (1993), which traces the role of gay men in relation to the course of the HIV epidemic in the west.

King recounts the details of the epidemiology of HIV and makes a strong case that informal peer education in gay communities was a major influence for containing HIV in the mid- to late-1980s, particularly in Britain (King, 1993: 37–84). With the advent of government health education campaigns aimed at the general population (and specifically *not* at gay men) and a lull in the incidence of activism within the gay community, HIV was allowed to increase again from the beginning of the 1990s (van den Hoek *et al.*, 1990). King's aim overtly is to make arguments for the provision of resources to gay men for HIV prevention. His arguments intentionally have a political slant, and could be criticized at times for selective use of empirical research findings, and not always distinguishing assumptions from deductions. It would, for example, be very difficult to *prove* that the British government's active inattention to gay men's health needs has 'had considerable harmful consequences for the sustenance of safer sex among gay men' (King, 1993: 188; no evidence is cited).

The interest here, however, is to focus on constructions of community and identity in the text. In this light, it appears that their meanings are slippery, and purposive, since they are used to make certain kinds of political claim. King discusses 'out' gay men (men who socially identify as gay) who use the commercial gay scene, deemed to be persons most at risk of contact with HIV in Britain (King, 1993: xii, 264). This might appear an easily defined group, yet there is no clear relationship of this description to a concept of community, nor who constitutes this group. The impression is given that 'we know who we're talking about': this means little more than 'people (assumed to be) like us'. Implicitly, though, 'out gay men' are treated as belonging to community in so far as they represent a community of sexual interest, an analysis arising from a tradition of gay activism in which sexual freedom was a key aim. King and other activists appear to follow Alcorn's distinction:

> In reality the lesbian and gay community has always been a network of communities, primarily split between a political community which pursues an ideal of political power and representation, and the communities of the night, which encompass the genuine diversity which political activists seek to represent.
>
> (Alcorn, 1992)

The activists argue that, since HIV is sexually transmitted, the aim of health promotion must be to reach the 'communities of the night' and, since these communities are *about* sex, eroticizing safer sex is an appropriate mode of action. As a counterpart to this, focusing on intimate relationships among gay men is seen as irrelevant, since 'romance' can lead to complacency about safer sex (Hardy, 1990), and reinforces heterosexist moralities of sex. The activist construction of community and its significance is thus radically different from Kayal's. It is sex-positive to the exclusion of other aspects of gay identity which may be significant to containing HIV.

Attached to the activist concern with community as community of sexual interest is a set of arguments about the distribution of resources, and the relation of out gay men to other men who have same gender sex. Out gay men on the commercial scene are deemed to be at highest risk for HIV because of the number of sexual partners they have and their likelihood of experiencing contexts in which unsafe sex is possible (King, 1993: 248). Resources for promoting and sustaining safer sex, therefore, must be made available to them, by Government, but through organisations of gay men working for gay men (King, 1993: 204, 264).

The analytical construct Men Who Have Sex With Men (MSM), as used, for example, by the Health Education Authority (1991), is seen as limiting and inappropriate, since, whilst intended to include men at risk for HIV who do not socially identify as gay, it is an alienating term for out gay men (who see it as clinical and authoritarian) and not a term that anyone else uses to identify themselves. So, it is argued, gay men should look after the interests of gay men. But where does this leave those other men who have sex with men, terminologically and practically? The activist argument is that hard to reach, sexually marginal men connect with out gay men sexually. Gay men are, therefore, the best placed people to convey safer sex information to them. A more radical version of this argument maintains that since a proud gay identity is most likely to sustain safer sex through high self-esteem, sexually marginal men can best be served by bringing them into community, by creating the conditions in which an out gay identity can be adopted (a large project indeed, because of its social structural and political implications; see Watney, 1993: 23). This is one of the aims of the organization GMFA. While such an argument appears to be logical, it returns us to the question of theorizing identity and community.

Ethnography, Identity and HIV/AIDS: Future Directions

The problem with the community proselytization argument is that it casts its net narrowly in terms of community as community of sexual interest. Men who have sex with men who are not out gay men is indeed a ridiculous classification, except for epidemiologists. Such men may also be husbands, fathers, bank managers, rock climbers, pimps and kleptomaniacs (amongst other things). It seems reasonable to assume that their primary identities may not be sexual (in a social sense at least). Who they are, and how best they can be involved in health promotion, are open questions. Ethnographic, anthropological research may have a role to play here. Such studies are usually based in concrete social contexts and take the view that all aspects of culture have to be seen relationally. A rounded ethnography looks at social actors in all their manifestations, and may therefore point to contexts in which safer sex education may happen. Richard Parker, discussing Brazil, shows how apprehending culturally specific 'erotic scripts' is essential for understanding when, how, and with whom specific sexual practices can be discussed (Parker, 1992). At the same time, good ethnography can contextualize sexuality as an aspect of identity, variable for different people and circumstances, avoiding a limiting focus on sexuality in itself and as an exclusionary theme. In this vein Cornwall and Lindisfarne's *Dislocating Masculinity* (1994) is a noteworthy contribution, deconstructing concepts of masculinity and illustrating, through diverse ethnographies, how masculinity is context-bound and tied to other aspects of identity, including gender and sexuality.

Though ethnographies may make use of key informants (such as AIDS activists with high public profiles), they are also about what is being said by those who do not feature in the media. This is important where activists are claiming to represent a very broad constituency. It would be informative, for example, to compare Kayal's cohort of AIDS volunteers (out gay men) with the client population they serve (persons who are HIV positive). In what precise senses are they the same people?

A gap unfortunately remains between academic and activist analyses. Kayal theorizes community in a sophisticated if controversial way without being able to operationalize these insights (beyond the example of GMHC) for enhancing HIV prevention. King has plenty of ideas for operationalizing prevention, but based on an under-theorized vision of community. In terms of HIV prevention, compromise and dialogue is evidently needed: one can theorize *ad infinitum* and partisan representations about HIV can hinder as well as help the aim of minimizing HIV in society as a whole.

Those of us who are social scientists and also gay men working on HIV/ AIDS might have an important role in mediating between activist concerns and areas of our work that may influence government policy. We bear responsibility toward other gay men (if we believe in 'gay community' at all), and should promote gay men's interests from our positions of relative power; yet as academics we also have a duty to detect and reject bullshit. Ralph Bolton's plea (1992) that participant observation in sex research should mean fucking your respondents (i.e. creating a concrete context for safer sex education) may be taking things a bit far, but this sort of provocation is necessary if academics are to be seen as doing more than observing through the keyhole. The signs are hopeful. The kind of dialogue proposed is happening in Britain through the annual Social Aspects of AIDS conference series, and smaller groupings such as the Gay Men's Workers' Forum in London. But these activities require wider and fuller development: complacency is the worst enemy.

References

ALCORN, K. (1992) 'Communities of the night', *Capital Gay*, 18 September.

ALTMAN, D. (1986) *AIDS and the New Puritanism*, London: Pluto Press.

APPLEBY, G.A and SOSNOWITZ, B.G. (1987) 'From social movement to social organization: Voluntary AIDS projects in Connecticut', paper presented at the Convention of the Society for the Study of Social Problems, Chicago, August.

ARNO, P. (1986) 'The nonprofit sector's response to the AIDS epidemic: Community-based services in San Francisco', *American Journal of Public Health*, **76**(11), 1325–30.

ARNO, P. (1988) 'The future of volunteerism and the AIDS epidemic', in ROGERS, D.E. and GINZBERG, E. (Eds.) *The AIDS Patient: An Action Agenda*, Boulder: Westview Press.

BABCHUK, N., MARSEY, R. and GORDON C.W. (1960) 'Men and women in community agencies: A note on power and prestige', *American Sociological Review*, **25**, 647–55.

BAYER, R. (1989) *Private Acts, Social Consequences: AIDS and the Politics of Public Health*, New York: Free Press, Macmillan.

BEESON, D., JONES, J.S. and NYE, J. (1986) 'The social consequences of AIDS antibody testing: Coping with stigma', paper presented at the 1986 Annual Meeting of the Society for the Study of Social Problems, New York.

BERRIDGE, V. and STRONG, P. (1992) 'AIDS policies in the United Kingdom: a preliminary analysis', in FEE, E. and FOX, D.M. (Eds) *AIDS: The Making of a Chronic Disease*, Berkeley: University of California Press.

BOLTON, R. (1992) 'Mapping terra incognita: Sex research for AIDS prevention – An urgent agenda for the 1990s', in HERDT, G. and LINDENBAUM, S. (Eds) *The Time of AIDS*, London: Sage.

CHAMBERS, C.A. (1985) 'The historical role of the voluntary sector in human service delivery in urban America', in TOBIN, G.A. (Ed.) *Social Planning and Human Service Delivery in the Voluntary Sector*, Westport, CN: Greenwood Press.

CHAMBRE, S.M. (1991) 'Volunteers as witnesses: The mobilization of AIDS volunteers in New York City, 1981–88', *Social Science Review*, **December**, 531–47.

CORNWALL, A. and LINDISFARNE, N. (1994) (Eds) *Dislocating Masculinity: Comparative Ethnographies*, London: Routledge.

CRIMP, D. (Ed.) (1988) *AIDS: Cultural Analysis, Cultural Activism*, Boston: MIT Press.

DAVIES P.M. (1987) 'Some problems in defining and sampling non-hetersexual males', London: Project SIGMA, Working Paper 3.

DAVIES, P. and PROJECT SIGMA, (1992) 'On relapse: recidivism or rational response?', in AGGLETON, P., DAVIES, P. and HART, G. (Eds) *AIDS: Rights, Risk and Reason*, London: Falmer Press.

DAVIES, P.M., WEATHERBURN, P., HUNT, A.J., HICKSON, F.C.I., McMANUS, T.J. and COXON, A.P.M. (1992) 'The sexual behaviour of young gay men in England and Wales', *AIDS Care*, **4**(3), 259–72.

DOWSETT, G., DAVIS, M. and CONNELL, R.W. (1992) 'Gay men, HIV/AIDS and social research: an Antipodean perspective', in AGGLETON, P. DAVIES, P. and HART, G. (Eds) *AIDS: Rights, Risk and Reason*, London: Falmer Press.

EARICKSON, R.J. (1990) 'International behavioural responses to a health hazard: AIDS', *Social Science and Medicine*, **31**(9), 851–962.

EDER, K. (1985) 'The new social movements: Moral crusades, political pressure groups, or social movements?', *New Social Research*, **52**, 869–90.

FITZPATRICK, R., HART, G., BOULTON, M., McLEAN, J. and DAWSON, J. (1989) 'Heterosexual sexual behaviour in a sample of homosexually active males', *Genito-Urinary Medicine*, **65**, 259–62.

FOUCAULT, M. (1977) *Discipline and Punish: The Birth of the Prison*, London: Allen Lane.

GAMSON, J. (1989) 'Silence, death and the invisible enemy: AIDS activism and social movement "Newness"', *Social Problems*, **36**(4), 351–67.

HABERMAS, J. (1981) 'New social movements', *Telos*, **49**, 33–7.

HARDY, R. (1990) 'Risky business: confronting unsafe sex', *Village Voice*, 26 June, 35–8.

HEALTH EDUCATION AUTHORITY (1991) *MESMAC: First Report.*, London: HEA.

HOLLERAN, A. (1987) 'Trust', *Christopher Street*, **10**(9), 4–8.

KATOFF, L. and DUNNE, R. (1988) 'Supporting people with AIDS: The gay men's health crisis model', *Journal of Palliative Care*, , 88–95.

KAYAL, P.M. (1986) 'The religious factor in AIDS', paper presented at the Society for the Scientific Study of Religion, Washington DC, 14 November.

KAYAL, P.M. (1993) *Bearing Witness: Gay Men's Health Crisis and the Politics of AIDS*, Boulder: Westview Press.

KING, E. (1993) *Safety in Numbers*, London: Cassell.

KIPPAX, S., CRAWFORD, J., CONNELL, R.W., DOWSETT, G.W., WATSON, L., RODDEN, P. *et al.* (1992) 'The importance of gay community in the prevention of HIV transmission: a study of Australian men who have sex with men', in AGGLETON, P., DAVIES, P. and HART, G. (Eds) *AIDS: Rights, Risk and Reason*, London: Falmer Press.

KIPPAX, S., CONNELL, R.W., DOWSETT, G. and CRAWFORD, J. (1993) *Sustaining Safe Sex*, London: Taylor & Francis.

KOBASA, S.C.O. (1990) 'AIDS and Volunteer Associations: Perspectives on Social and Individual Change', *Millbank Quarterly*, **68** (Suppl 2) , 280–94.

OFFE, C. (1985) 'The new social movements: Challenging the boundaries of institutional politics', *Social Research*, **52**(4), 817–68.

PARKER, R. (1992) 'Sexual diversity, cultural analysis, and AIDS education in Brazil', in HERDT, G. and LINDENBAUM, S. (Eds) *The Time of AIDS*, London: Sage.

POLLAK, M., PAICHELER, G. and PIERRET, J. (1992) *AIDS: A Problem for Sociological Research*, London: Sage.

SCOTT, P. (1992) 'Wake up! Fight back!', *Capital Gay*, **545**, 22 May.

TOURAINE, A. (1985) 'An introduction to the study of social movements', *Social Research*, **52**(4), 749–87.

VAN DEN HOEK, J.A.R., VAN GRIENSVEN, G.J.P. and COUTINHO, R.A. (1990) 'Increase in unsafe homosexual behaviour', *The Lancet*, **336**, 179—80.

WATNEY, S. (1993) 'Emergent sexual identities and HIV/AIDS', in AGGLETON, P., HART, G. and DAVIES, P. (Eds) *AIDS: Facing the Second Decade*, London: Falmer Press.

WEATHERBURN, P., DAVIES, P.M., HUNT, A.J., COXON, A.P.M. and MCMANUS, T.J. (1990) 'Heterosexual behaviour in a large cohort of homosexually active men in England and Wales', *AIDS Care*, **2**(4), 319–24.

WEEKS, J. (1986) *Sexuality*, London: Routledge.

WEITZ, R. (1989) *Life with AIDS*, New Brunswick: Rutgers University Press.

Chapter 12

Sexuality, Identity and Community – Reflections on the MESMAC Project

Katie Deverell and Alan Prout

This chapter reflects on some of the issues that arose out of a particular HIV-related project called MESMAC. We were the evaluators of this project and we use some of the material gathered in the research to analyse how aspects of sexuality, identity and community came into play and interacted with each other during the project's work. Through a discussion of this material we then raise questions about the adequacy and use of concepts such as sexuality, community and identity. In the final part of the chapter we suggest the need for alternative ways of looking at identity that capture better its often shifting and flexible character. In particular we suggest the importance of a focus on the social processes by which individuals and groups construct and deconstruct their identities as significant 'facts'. We relate this to the potential usefulness of the broader and more flexible concept of 'affinity' suggested by writers such as Haraway (1990). We feel that a consideration of such issues is not just theoretically interesting but of practical importance to HIV prevention.

Background to MESMAC

First, we describe what MESMAC was (for a fuller account see Prout and Deverell, 1995). MESMAC is an acronym for Men Who Have Sex with Men – Action in the Community. It was a three-year community development project funded by the Health Education Authority (HEA). It comprised four sites in different parts of England (London, Leicester, Leeds and Newcastle-upon-Tyne), which were linked together by a national structure. Each site had a general brief to work with men who have sex with men (MWHSWM) in relation to HIV, safer sex and other health needs, and a more specific brief of its own. It was continuously evaluated throughout these three years by ourselves working collaboratively with the members of the local and national project teams.

The project arose from a decision within the HEA to set up an HIV-prevention project that took a collective action approach, rather than the more usual focus on individual behaviour change. The particular type of collective action chosen for MESMAC was Community Development or CD.[1] In retrospect it seems clear that the project was constituted within a fundamental tension: as a CD project it was rooted in the idea of working within the context of community; at the same time it incorporated terminology based around sexual practice rather than identity. Thus, the community towards whom the project was targeted was not defined in community terms at all. This tension was well captured by one of the project workers:

> I think there are some issues about fitting a CD model to MWHSWM really, in as much as that MWHSWM is about an activity, whereas CD is about identity, in a lot of ways about society, about groups and about communities. So it feels very difficult, how to use a CD model with someone who doesn't have any social, political networks with other gay men, or other MWHSWM, and will they be artificial constructs if you try to put that together?
>
> (Interview, 29.7.92)

At the outset it was clear that CD was at least feasible as a way of working with gay men but it was not at all clear whether or how community development might work with behaviourally defined MWHSWM. The project, therefore, was involved in a complex exploration of the relationship between community, identity and behaviour. Its strength lay exactly in its commitment to work with these two, at times contradictory, notions.

Sexual Identity

It has now been well established that all sexual identities are historically specific, contingent, constructed and changing (Watney, 1993; Weeks, 1986). As Padgug has argued:

> Homosexual and 'heterosexual' behaviour may be universal; homosexual and heterosexual identity and consciousness are modern realities. These identities are not inherent in the individual. In order to be gay, for example, more than individual inclinations (however we might conceive of those) or homosexual activity is required; entire ranges of social attitudes and the construction of particular cultures,

subcultures, and social relations are first necessary. To 'commit' a homosexual act is one thing; to be a homosexual is something entirely different.

(Padgug, 1989: 60)

For some time the social constructionist approach[2] to sexuality has highlighted how physically identical sexual acts may have varying social significance and subjective meaning depending on how they are defined and understood in different cultures and historical periods (Vance, 1991). For example, as Alonso and Kopreck have written in relation to their work with Mexican MWHSWM:

> ... Anglo-American sexual distinctions-'heterosexual', 'bisexual', and 'homosexual' ... are neither universal nor natural but instead socioculturally and historically produced categories which cannot be presumed to be applicable to US minority groups or to other societies.
>
> (Alonso and Kopreck,1993: 114)

Such research has shown that the relationship between sexual practices and the meanings attached to them is not fixed. This has led to a formulation of sexuality as composed of sexual identity, sexual practice and sexual desire with a recognition that there is no necessary connection between these elements (Patton, 1985). However, it is recognized that in the lives of individuals sexual identity is often thought of as if it were a direct, unmediated product of sexual desire (Rust, 1993). As Vance has argued, understanding the ways in which sexual categories are produced at the level of culture and history:

> Does not mean that individuals have an open-ended ability to construct themselves multiple times in adulthood. (This is not to deny individuals' experiences of sexual malleability and change, which are probably considerably more extensive than our cultural frames and our own biographical narratives admit.)
>
> (Vance, 1989: 17)

MESMAC drew on social constructionist theories of sexuality incorporating the then fashionable terminology MWHSWM because of its recognition that there is no necessary link between sexual identity and sexual behaviour. Thus, for example, a man may have sex with another man but not define himself as gay or bisexual. For an HIV project this was seen as important as men may be placing themselves at risk through specific sexual practices but not reached by, or relate to, campaigns focused around identity.

The experience of MESMAC reinforced the view that MWHSWM are a diverse group, and that there is no clear relationship between sexual identity and practice. For example, some men contacted by the project identified as gay or bisexual and were known as such by friends and family; others self-identified as gay or bisexual but were not known to be so by others. Others did not have a definite sexual identity: many of the married men and some of the rent boys contacted by the project expressed feeling confused about their sexuality. Some of these men went on to define themselves as gay or bisexual, whilst others did not. Still others felt the identities available to them were not culturally appropriate, or did not feel a need to have a sexual identity.[3] As one of the MESMAC workers explained:

> My experience of the majority of the people we've worked with on the streets is that a lot of the men didn't have sexual identities, nor did they feel the need for one, you know and it was us who was attributing it and we were defining their sexuality in terms of sexual practice which is you know, that's just not on
>
> (Interview, 29.7.92)

This lack of need for an identity based on sexual practice has also been reported in an Australian context by Bartos, McLeod and Nott. They state that for many non-identifying MWHSWM, sexual identity is largely irrelevant:

> Sexual identity is not a major issue for msm (men who have sex with men). Sexuality is not a key part of their sense of personal identity, which is based instead on other personal relationships (e.g. family, career etc.)
>
> (Bartos *et al.*, 1993: iv)

The experience of MESMAC and other projects suggests that it is a mistake to assume that all MWHSWM have an identity constructed around their sexual practice. Even when men contacted by MESMAC did have a clear sexual identity, this was not always revealing about their sexual behaviour. For example, men identifying as gay might be having sex with women, and men who identified as straight might be having sex with men. This complex situation reinforced the lack of necessary commensurability between identity and practice that is well documented in sexuality and sex research literature, and has been raised by numerous other MWHSWM projects (Bartos *et al.*, 1993; Boulton and Weatherburn, 1990; BMRB,1992; Davies, 1990; Davis *et al.*, 1991; Murray, 1992;Prestage and Hood, 1993; Rodden *et al.*, 1993; Siegel and Bauman, 1986; Weatherburn *et al.*, 1992).

This situation highlights the complexity of how people choose to identify themselves; people may share the same sexual practices but identify in different ways, or choose not to build an identity relating to their sexual practice. This is an important point. It has recently been argued by some gay men critiquing the use of the term MWHSWM that 'In reality, they (MWHSWM) either identify as heterosexual or bisexual' (Watney, 1993:23).

Some critics have gone on to suggest that the term 'gay, bisexual or other' should be used. Whilst recognizing some difficulties with the term MWHSWM, the experience of MESMAC is that returning to the use of categories such as bisexual is an oversimplification of the situation. Contrary to the idea that MWHSWM either identify as gay or bisexual, some MWHSWM do not profess having a sexual identity at all, or have not thought about their sexual practice in this way. In any case, there may be vast differences between men who choose to identify as bisexual and those who are defined by others as behaviourally bisexual, indeed the latter category would also include some gay identified men.

Identity, Community and Collective Action

One of the early experiences of the project was that it was easier to work collectively with men who had open and confident gay identities (this also has been reported by Davis *et al.* (1991) in an Australian context). Workers found it particularly hard to collectivise work with men who did not positively identify as gay or bisexual, or who wanted to keep their identity secret. It is instructive in this respect that Patton, describing the work of D'Emilio, Weeks and Bronski in relation to the development of modern gay identities and communities, notes that:

> Each views the development of a *public* [our emphasis] sexual identification as a key stage in the process of identity and community formation.
>
> (Patton, 1985: 123)

Indeed, MESMAC workers found that it was much easier to develop collective action with those men who were willing to be out about their sexual identity. This underlines an important difference with much other CD work that is organized around identities, issues or communities that are public, or with which people are happy to be associated, for example their place of residence. Many MWHSWM do not have a public sexual identity, or indeed do not want an identity based around their sexual practice. This makes immediate collective action more difficult as work usually has to proceed in ways that will not publicly identify them, limiting the kind of activities that can be undertaken.

The project workers found that many MWHSWM who did not identify as gay were resistant to the forms of collective action they attempted to facilitate, and were only interested in accessing resources, support and information. One of the main reasons for this was that for many men, having sex with other men was something that they kept secret. For these men, the prospect of working collectively ran the risk of their being identified as a MWHSWM, or involved being open about their activities in a way that was totally unacceptable and unrealistic. For example, workers found that much of sex in public sex environments was silent and that even trying to make contact with some of the men here was impossible. Most of the men contacted in these places did not feel part of a community and had no desire to collectivize their experience, often the sexual activity was all they wanted. As one of the workers explained:

> ... what they do is about sex, it genuinely is about sex, it's not about wanting anything else and not being able to get it. It's not about wanting to be gay, wanting a relationship, wanting to come out etc., those men are quite happy as they are.'
>
> (Interview, 24.2.92)

It was important that this was respected and that it was not assumed that all MWHSWM wanted to come out and adopt a gay identity (see also Bartos *et al.*, 1993; Prestage and Hood, 1993).

The majority of the workers in MESMAC were gay identified men and, for many, a primary motivation for being involved in MESMAC was to do work with gay men. Because of their own strong gay identity, a difficulty for some of the workers lay in accepting that not all MWHSWM wanted to identify as gay. Many of the workers wanted to support men coming out and validate their gay identity (see also Davis *et al.*, 1991). However, as work progressed they realised that the situation was more complex. Many of the MWHSWM did not see themselves as gay, or did not want to take on this identity. Workers felt that as out gay men they may alienate some men who have sex with men. This was of particular concern in outreach work where it was clear that some MWHSWM shied away from contact with gay identified men. As a worker said:

> ... one of my concerns is the difficulty of having to target MWHSWM ... who maybe have a strong heterosexual identity, as a very out, gay worker ... [for] someone who has no contact with the gay world apart from a bit of sex on the side ... To be confronted with someone who is very out, and is coming from that point of view may be completely alien and off putting. It's very effective when you want to go to a [gay] club, it's brilliant, but outside that environment it has a down side.
>
> (Interview, 29.7.92)

Indeed, many of the black men whom the Leicester project met in saunas drew a distinction between themselves as MWHSWM (or 'MESMEN', to use the term invented by the Leicester project workers), and gay men whom they did not identify with. As a worker said: 'Mesmen will often distinguish between what they do, that is, have sex with men and what gay men do, which is love men, be camp, live together etc.' (Interview, 10.3.92). For these men, the value of MESMAC lay in the opportunity to access resources and support without having to identify as gay or bisexual. This experience underlines the importance of developing a more detailed understanding of the complexity of identity. Although writers such as Simon Watney are right to point out that homophobia has a huge impact on the choices people feel able to make about their sexual identities, the experience of MESMAC is that it is wrong to assume that all MWHSWM are somewhere along a road which is clearly moving towards a gay identity. Thus it is not a case, as Watney has argued, that the correct response to the question of men whose behaviour may be asymmetrical with their sexual identity is to combat and minimize the powerful obstacles to their obtaining a gay identity (Watney, 1993: 23) but to recognize men's different needs and desires in relation to a specifically sexual identity.

Within MESMAC it did prove possible, if done sensitively, to form groups for (or including) non-gay identified men by focusing on issues other than sexual identity. For example, Rent Boy Action in Leeds (a self-help group for rent boys) focused around legal rights and dealing with harassment. Workers also encouraged individual men to become involved in particular groups of interest to them. Although it was recognized that collective action was not always appropriate in relation to non-identifying MWHSWM (outreach, phone work and one-to-one work being preferable), for some men this was important. For those who wanted it, the opportunity to meet, talk with and get support from other men was very valuable, particularly in reducing isolation and reassuring men that others were in a similar situation.

As mentioned above, for those men who had a sexual identity, and who were open about it, collective work was significantly easier. This was often the case as many gay identified men became involved as a way of supporting other gay men or to share their experiences with others (King, 1993). The process of sharing experiences and working collectively, of being put in touch with other groups and organizations, of making new friends, and being able to develop their own initiatives was of great importance. It helped many of those who became involved to feel a strengthened sense of community. For some men, such contact with the project led to a greater certainty and confidence in their own sexual identity, which led to a decision to come out. This way of working also showed evidence of men adopting and maintaining safer sex, through promoting self-esteem and strengthening attachment to the gay community and gay identity (see also King, 1993; Kippax *et al.*, 1990).

However, working around shared identity was not always easy. Not all gay men were out and so they were still put off by the thought of being discovered. Other men were just coming out and as such found the prospect of going to a gay group intimidating; as one MESMAC user said 'even going to a gay group is like coming out'. In addition some gay men felt that having a common identity did not focus enough; and some felt that there were other identities they would rather organize around.

Although MESMAC has shown that it is much easier to attract men to groups if they share something in common, this 'thing' may be additional to their sexuality. Often, sexual identity is not enough, or rather other differences can be more important than a shared sexual identity. Some of the longest-running MESMAC groups were those based on specific activities that were additional to gay identity and provided an organizing focus. An example was the lesbian and gay theatre group 'Latex Productions' (see Deverell and Doyle, 1992). This does not mean that sexual identity is not important, but on its own it is not always sufficient as a focus for organization. Other differences and experiences such as class, race or political views can fracture any unity based on shared sexual identity.

Within MESMAC, recognition of this diversity and complexity highlighted the limitations of using categories based on identity. However, the workers had particular flexibility because the CD strategy emphasized working with men on the basis of the needs they themselves expressed and prioritized, rather than those they were assumed to have. This legitimized specific initiatives for men who were having sex with men but who did not necessarily identify as gay or who could be reached as, for example, black men, married men or rent boys.

Who Defines Identity?

A key issue that arose in the course of the project related to the process of identification and the fact that identity is not automatic. By this we mean that how people choose to identify themselves cannot be assumed; even if people choose to identify in certain ways this may not always be accepted by others. For example, some of the gay identified rent boys said that many gay men looked down upon them, or made it clear that they did not want rent boys to be associated with the gay community. Thus, not all self-identified gay men were seen to be part of the community and some felt excluded by it. Organizing work around identity and community therefore could have the disadvantage of reproducing existing inequalities related to race, ability, class, occupation, age and other social divisions. This issue has been pointed out by other commentators in relation to earlier grassroots work around safer sex (Altman, 1988; Dada, 1990; Patton, 1990) and is supported by MESMAC's experience. For example, deaf gay men and black men contacted by the project have argued strongly that they have missed out on previous information and support, or that available services, information and support have been inappropriate or inaccessible. A good example of this is provided by the fact that at the time the project started, the workers could find no existing British HIV-prevention posters featuring black gay men. This raises the important point of who is seen as being gay, or belonging to the gay community, and suggests that some identities are not equally available to all.

One of the practical issues that arose from the fact that identity is not necessarily obvious and automatic lay in deciding who it was appropriate for the project to contact. For example, although in outreach work there were various signs that the workers could pick up on, attempting to identify which men it would be appropriate to talk to was often very complicated (see Deverell, 1992). As one worker explained talking about his outreach work in a sauna:

> ... it is really difficult 'cos one week you might think 'Hmm he's straight'. The next week you might think 'Oh he must be gay' ... It goes backwards and forwards it's really quite strange. It's quite nice to see actually, because it tells you a lot about people and the way people act, but it's confusing as well and it's hard to actually go up to someone and say 'Oh I actually work for MESMAC' 'cos you don't know how safe you are.
>
> (Interview, 12.12.90)

Similar experiences to those of the MESMAC workers have also been reported for outreach work with (behaviourally) bisexual men in Australia, as Davis *et al.* write:

> Often a worker's supposition about the type of man he is approaching is wrong. For example, the worker initially decided to approach men with wedding rings and who looked straight, in an effort to talk to bisexually active men. However, many of these men said they were gay and had no sexual relationships with women. At other times a man assumed to be gay and with very typical patterns of social interaction in the gay community was also having sex with women.
>
> (Davis *et al.*, 1991: 7–8)

Workers learnt to observe very closely and to keep an open mind when observing people. All of the workers spoke of the need to err on the side of caution when approaching people, with some suggesting that this led them to target certain men.

Another related issue arose for black workers who found that some service users did not identify themselves as black, or felt they had little in common with other black men and therefore actually preferred to talk to white workers. Some black men were also in relationships with white partners and worried about alienating them through becoming involved in a black project. The situation was made more difficult because the workers found that by concentrating their efforts on targeting black men, many men assumed that the project was political rather than there to provide a service. As a worker explained: 'Because you have black in your title you become a pressure group rather than a service provider' (Interview, 214.6.91). This meant that the work attained an additional political dynamic. The workers felt that black men sometimes shied away from contact with the project because of this. For others there was a fear of being identified as a MWHSWM. This meant that some men felt threatened by the approach of someone from the same community. As one of the workers reported: 'Asian men will come to the door (of the sauna) and ask if other Asian men are there, if there are they don't come in' (Interview, 3.11.92). This experience underlines the importance of not making assumptions about how people choose to identify themselves, or who they will feel most comfortable with.

One of the important considerations in relation to work with black men was the need to address the complexity of identity and to recognize that people may choose to identify themselves in different ways. For example, some black men said there was a need for more black men to come out and identify as gay, and for there to be greater visibility of black, gay role models. However, others questioned the need for a gay identity, which they saw as a white, western one. Many black MWHSWM did not (and did not want to) define themselves as gay. A very important finding in the London and Leicester work was that many of the black men using the scene had female partners. Leicester estimated that about 75 per cent of the men that they worked with were married, or had relationships with female partners. Gay identified material, therefore, was often inappropriate, or seen as offensive, and only met some of the needs that these men had. Indeed, MESMAC found that most black MWHSWM do not relate to HIV prevention if it is organized around gay identity. There was a need, therefore, to support black MWHSWM who did not want to take on a gay identity, as well as those who chose to identify as gay. Workers had to be sensitive to the different experiences and lifestyles of black MWHSWM and to work from the basis of men's self-identity.

Multiplicity of Identity

Another of the important practical experiences in the work was the need to recognize that men may have more than one identity, and attachment to various communities. In particular, the work with black men highlighted the need for a more complex understanding of the interplay of race and sexuality on people's identities. For some men, their sexual identity was not always the most prominent or important identity. For example, in a racist society many black men may experience more need for social support around race than sexuality. This is particularly the case since black men are more likely to be identified and discriminated against on the basis of race. This means that many black MWHSWM are more likely to get involved in, and take action around the social and political issues affecting black communities, rather than organize around sexuality.

This situation was not unique to black men, many of the issues also arose in MESMAC work with South East Asian and Jewish men. It was also true of white men. For example, at times their age, class or occupation could be more important than their sexuality. Workers had to come to terms with the fact that sexuality could not be separated out from other aspects of people's identities and lives. As one worker said:

> My own experience of talking to white gay men is that black gay feelings are marginalized and dismissed, (it's either) 'We're all gay, we all feel the same', or they've never thought about it ... often when you are thinking of coming out there isn't really a great deal to attract you ... The whole of the gay scene as I know it isn't particularly geared towards black people. You can't think 'I'll come out because I'll have lots of support, lots of people to help me bear the pressures etc.' I'm all for making black people more comfortable (with their sexuality) rather than coming out totally isolated, or finding the only support they have is of a sexual nature.
>
> (Interview, 8.5.91)

MESMAC has shown that people have different identities that are more or less important in relation to different situations, times and people (see also Gatter, 1991, 1993; Weeks, 1990). This means that it is important to understand identity as a more fluid and shifting phenomenon. For some men, their identity at a specific moment seems to have been related to the social context within which they were speaking. For example, the project workers in Leeds, who have strong and proud identities as gay men, reported that sex workers mostly identify as gay when in conversation with them. In contrast, one of the key figures in Rent Boy Action, himself a gay identified man and an ex-rent boy, said that when working on the streets rent boys mostly claimed to be straight. The point here is not that one or the other identity must be true, but just the opposite – that sexual identity may be more fluid and that it arises and is formed in a context.

This fluidity of identity, or at least the fact that different identities are important at different times was a clear finding in the relation to work with black men. Peterson (1992) writing on the experiences of black gay men in America, has suggested that there are two types of men: 'black gays' and 'gay blacks'. He argues that:

> Black gay men are more likely to base their self-identity on their race

than on their sexual orientation. In comparison, 'gay blacks' may be described as men whose allegiance is affected more by their sexual orientation than their race, who are more likely to be open about their homosexual identity, and who are often involved in the white gay community.

(Peterson, 1992: 153–4)

Contrary to this view, the black workers in MESMAC suggested that rather than seeing these black men as different types, it was more important to consider the context within which men's different identities were asserted. These workers themselves felt that sometimes they identified more strongly as black at other times more as gay men. However, even this conception of identity is in some ways insufficient as identities cannot be neatly separated out from each other. As Avtar Brah has written:

Structures of class, racism, gender and sexuality cannot be treated as 'independent variables' because the oppression of each is inscribed within the other – is constituted by and is constitutive of the other.

(Brah, 1992: 137)

Thus, it is not simply a case of thinking about race and thinking about sexuality and trying to fit these issues together, but considering how race and sexuality interact and affect each other. For example, the way ideas about race construct black men's sexuality as exotic and animalistic (Manuel *et al.* 1989; see also Brake, 1976 on gender and sexuality; Rutherford, 1990). It is important that the multiplicity of identity is not seen in a simplistic, additive way.

The multiplicity of identity underlines another important point, that gay men themselves have different understandings of the notion of a gay identity and do not attach equal importance to it (Plummer, 1975). For example, some men, though identifying as gay, do not feel that they have much in common with other gay men. This means that sexual identity has different meanings for different people and as such it is not necessarily a unifying factor. Therefore, although having a gay identity can be an important unifying focus for some men, it is important to consider the costs of only working in this way; it may serve to exclude those who choose not to define as such, or indeed define themselves in opposition to gay men. Work that appeals only to gay identity and community, though important, will not reach many other men who have sex with men.

It is important that this fluidity of identity is taken into account. Identities are not fixed and unitary but multiple, historical and contingent. Workers have to be flexible and acknowledge that men may choose to identify, or are identified, in different ways at different times.

Structural Aspects of Identity

As we have suggested above, identity is not just an individual choice/essence but arises from a process of interaction within social contexts. As Rust argues:

> Social constructionism teaches that self-identity is the result of the interpretation of personal experience in terms of available social constructs. Identity is therefore a reflection of sociopolitical organization rather than a reflection of essential organization.
>
> (Rust, 1993: 68)

This means that different choices are available to people depending on how they relate to the current social constructs. For example, a further consideration in the work with black men related to their choices around coming out. Obviously, for many white men coming out can be a difficult and painful process and there is often a hard choice to be made between family and sexuality, with many men leaving their families to come out. Many black men find this choice is somewhat less clear cut. For example, for many black men the family is one of the few places where they can get support from racism. Additionally, it is a place where they can draw on and experience their own culture and traditions, as opposed, for example, to a predominantly white, European gay scene. The Leicester workers found that many of the black MWHSWM they met were disillusioned with the scene. They had high expectations of it as a place where they would be accepted and get support but instead had felt isolated and marginalized. Because the lesbian and gay community appears to be so white and the scene is often racist and alienating, black men could feel that coming out and entering the gay community would be more difficult than staying at home and keeping their sexual identity secret. As Peterson describes:

> Faced with anti-gay attitudes in the black community and anti-black attitudes in the gay community, black gay men experience a severe conflict between their racial identity and their sexual orientation.
>
> (Peterson, 1992: 150)

Therefore, as one of the workers pointed out:

> Moving away from the family is a bigger deal. It is the only place I feel completely comfortable. I can get support, speak patois, eat Jamaican food, there are lots of other ties.
>
> (Interview, 21.2.93)

Some Asian married men also reported that they received financial support from their families in return for keeping to cultural norms. This meant that coming out or making their sexuality known entailed a possible additional cost. This was particularly the case because coming out as gay could damage the marriage prospects of their brothers and sisters. Many black men felt that their identity was more bound up with their families than is the case for a lot of white men (similar experiences have been reported for Chicano men in Latin America (see Almaguer 1993)).

MESMAC workers described how many black men felt they were in limbo, stuck between two worlds, neither of which would accept them completely. Although many white men do not feel comfortable on the gay scene, and many white families are not accepting of homosexuality either, white men may be able to find more support amongst the lesbian and gay community. These experiences underline how structural and cultural factors influence the choices people feel able to make about their identity (see also Almaguer, 1993).

Sexual Identity of the Workers

The sexual identity of the workers proved to be a great asset in the development of the work, with many gay identified users commenting that it helped to build trust, as well as provide a feeling of empathy and under-standing. Generally, it was felt that it was best to employ gay men to do work with gay men. However, it was important to recognize that being gay did not necessarily mean that workers would have had similar experiences with users. Sometimes other differences such as class meant that they had very different life experiences and lifestyles (see Deverell and Prout, 1992). For this reason, the experience of MESMAC was that although it was important to have a majority of gay men working in a project for gay men, others may also have a useful contribution. As one project member said:

> I think there is a danger, and that's part of the sort of fascism that is around at the moment, that everything for gay men or MWHSWM has to be done by MWHSWM. I think that to a certain extent is outrageous, because I think whilst you need an overwhelming proportion of gay men to work in that area people should be entitled to have a choice, and people don't necessarily relate easily to other gay men who come from a particular standpoint about their gayness.
>
> (Interview, 4.11.92)

Indeed, within MESMAC many of the workers found personal difficulties in working with men who did not identify as gay. Furthermore, they did only a little work that addressed the sex that many of these men had with women (see also Davis *et al.*, 1991). For example, the Leeds team described how when working with Rent Boy Action, they always showed gay safer sex videos and would have felt uncomfortable with heterosexual materials, even though some of the men identified as straight or bisexual. They wondered whether this was one of the reasons why those men who stayed in the group either defined, or came to define themselves as gay. This view was supported by a member of Rent Boy Action who said:

> I mean our group's not specifically a gay group ... and so a lot of members don't want to know about gay issues, and like MESMAC's always wanting to push gay issues, well just gay sex or gay activities.
>
> (Interview, 13.2.93)

For those MWHSWM who were having sex with women, organizing work around gay communities and identities had the effect of only addressing part of their sexuality. For example, many of the men with female partners did not know about HIV-transmission routes between men and women, and having information that only addressed sex with men did not help this situation. As an HIV project, it was important that such issues were addressed, particularly as these were often of major concern to the men themselves, for example men wanted help in negotiating safer sex with female partners or in getting support to come out to them, or just wanted to talk about their relationships. It proved important not to assume that such issues only applied to men who identified as straight or bisexual, as gay identified men may also be having sex with women (see, for example, BMRB, 1992; Weatherburn *et al.*, 1992), a point that some commentators seem to overlook (Scott, 1993). In this respect, thinking about the community and identity boundaries that were worked within, was important. Men may be having sex with men who were seen to belong to different communities, or having sex which in the current orthodoxy would seem to place them in different communities. This highlights the practical importance of considering theoretical issues relating to the construction of sexuality, community and identity.

Conclusion: Identity, Fluidity and Affinity

So far we have discussed some of the experiences of MESMAC in relation to sexuality, identity and community. The experience of the project was that using a CD approach offered the ability and commitment to combine both the benefits of community-based work with the importance of recognizing and addressing diversity. By organizing work around sexual identity and community the projects worked successfully with existing community organizations and networks of gay and bisexual men. Building on this basis of shared experience and support proved particularly useful in collectivizing work. However, the work also identified a diversity of need and experience amongst MWHSWM, both within gay and bisexual communities, as well as amongst men who did not identify in these ways. This highlighted how an emphasis on community and commonality can also hide diversity. The experience of MESMAC is that there is a need to look beyond the boundaries of existing communities in order to reach MWHSWM who do not identify as gay or who feel marginalized from gay communities because of their age, race or differing commitment to a gay identity. In this case, successful collective work often involves organizing around something other than sexuality, and recognizing the diversity of men's identities. MESMAC has shown that a major challenge for HIV prevention is to come up with methods that can embrace the shifting, multiple and fragmentary nature of identity.

Up until this point in the discussion we have retained the term identity. However, it is clear from the examples we have highlighted that identity (as an individual or collectively as a community) is problematic. The experience of MESMAC has reinforced that identity is multiple, contested and contextual and shown that different identities are constructed by individuals and groups at different places and times. This has led us to consider more processual ways of thinking. As Stuart Hall has suggested in relation to Caribbean cultural identities:

> Identity is not as transparent or unproblematic as we think. Perhaps instead of thinking of identity as an already accomplished fact ... we should think, instead, of identity as a 'production', which is never complete, always in process, and always constituted within, not outside, representation.
>
> (Hall, 1990, 222)

Indeed, the 'fact' of an identity can be seen as dependent upon a large range of contingencies – just some of which are illustrated by our discussion of how these were encountered in the MESMAC project. This 'facticity' is not a given (of biology or anything else) but a constantly worked on, contested and fragile product. Furthermore, it seems clear that part of the work of producing identity as a fact includes bringing together possibly divergent social worlds. Seen in this way, establishing sexual identity involves trading-off against other identities drawn from other social worlds, for example in relation to class, religion or race. Sociologists of (scientific) knowledge have created the term 'boundary object' to describe this type of phenomenon. They state that:

> Boundary objects are both adaptable to different viewpoints and robust enough to maintain identity between them.
>
> (Star and Griesmer, 1989: 1)

The creation of boundary objects involves collective action '... managed across social worlds in order to achieve enough agreement to get work done and produce relatively (and temporarily) stable "facts"' (Fujimura, 1992). The process involves the creation of a framework within which actors from different social worlds can be brought together and held together for long enough and with a connection strong enough for something new to be created. The production of novel 'facts' is a sign that a boundary object has been successfully created. On the other hand, the attempt to connect social worlds often founders on sets of meanings being experienced as incommensurate and even incompatible.

The parallels with sexual identity as a produced fact are enlightening. In order to create an identity, its 'facticity' has to be worked at and established. This is achieved, for example, through the construction of (amongst others) shared histories, symbols, language and dress (see Butler, 1993: 310).

For many gay men and lesbians, the translation of their identity (as an individual or as a collectivity) into a fact is a vital political necessity. In the face of deep-rooted homophobia, the attempt is to forge solidarity on the basis of shared but not identical histories, structural positions and interests (Martin, 1993: 283). As Butler has written:

> But politically, we might argue, isn't it quite crucial to insist on lesbian and gay identities precisely because they are being threatened with erasure and obliteration from homophobic quarters? ... Isn't it 'no accident' that such theoretical contestations of identity emerge within a political climate that is performing a set of similar obliterations of homosexual identities through legal and political means?
>
> (Butler 1993: 311)

We do not wish to reproduce the invisibility of lesbians and gay men by questioning the importance of identity. However, we are aware (and have shown above) that for some MWHSWM the translation of their sexual desires and behaviour into the 'fact' of gay identity is not only difficult but may be strongly resisted. In addition, this potentially totalizing identity can serve to conceal important differences between gay men, and may make certain issues difficult to address. It is for this reason that we have begun to question the usefulness of identity as an analytical concept. A number of writers have also begun to move in the same direction, Martin, for example, points out that:

> ... A number of marginalized communities now face important questions about the possibility of reconceptualising identity without abandoning it and its strategic deployment altogether.
>
> (Martin,1993: 275)

It may be, however, that more radical solutions have to be sought. One way forward has been suggested by Dona Haraway writing in relation to feminism. Through the experience of the feminist movement, and in particular the writing of many black feminists, she has suggested that it is important to move away from totalizing identities and theories. She writes that:

Identities seem contradictory, partial, and strategic. With the hard-won recognition of their social and historical constitution, gender, race, and class cannot provide the basis for belief in 'essential' unity. There is nothing about being 'female' that naturally binds women. There is not even such a state as 'being' female, itself a highly complex category constructed in contested sexual scientific discourses and other social practices . . . Painful fragmentation among feminists (not to mention among women) along every possible fault line has made the concept of woman elusive . . . The recent history for much of the U.S. Left and the U.S. feminism has been a response to this kind of crisis by endless splitting and searches for a new essential unity. But there has also been a growing recognition of another response through coalition-affinity, not identity.

(Haraway, 1990: 197)

Haraway argues against relying on totalizing and essentialized identities, and suggests instead a move to the latter approach, that is, for responses based on affinity rather than identity (see also Alonso and Kopreck (1993). This involves recognizing that forms of identity and community are chosen, negotiated and achieved, not simply given. As Sandoval notes:

United States Third World feminists are pointing out the differences that exist among all women not in order to fracture any hope of unity among women but to propose a new order-one that provides a new possibility for unity without the erasure of differences. This new order would draw attention to the construction and ideological con-sequences of every order, of every community, of every identity.

(Sandoval, quoted in Martin, 1993: 283)

As a consequence of adopting the idea of affinity, the importance of building unities rather than naturalizing them is highlighted (Haraway, 1990). In this way the concept of affinity is reminiscent of alliance building and potentially feeds into ideas currently emerging from queer politics (see Berube and Escoffier, 1991).

MESMAC began by working within the tension between identity and behaviour. Through the frontline experience of its workers, and a structure which encouraged reflection on that experience, the practice of the project was closer to the sort of flexibility that the concept of affinity suggests.[4] The project succeeded in enabling a diversity of men to organize around issues defined, by themselves, as important. It recognized that this approach was more successful than expecting men to organize collectively around a sexual identity that they may or may not share. By recognizing the importance of differences rather than trying to subsume them under a necessarily prioritized gay identity, a greater diversity of men were able to be involved. This also meant that effort was put into building links and trying to enable men who had previously felt marginalized from the gay community to be involved.

By promoting the usefulness of the concept of affinity, we are far from suggesting that the notion of identity be entirely rejected. However, as a basis for collective action organizing work around the idea of affinity seems likely to lead to more flexible and creative alliances and to involve more sensitivity to the multiplicity of difference. In consequence more people will be able to participate in HIV-prevention initiatives than if these are organized around identity alone.

Notes

1   There are many different definitions of Community Development (CD) but they all share some important principles (see, for example, Martin, 1990; Sheffield Health Authority, 1993; Smithies, 1991). Indeed, CD is probably best thought of as a way of working, informed by certain principles, rather than the application of a particular method. Within MESMAC, the work was conducted around a specific CD strategy that stressed the need to work at several different levels. These levels were: *grass roots work* (such as outreach, starting new groups) to identify needs, build on shared experiences and promote new solutions to locally defined problems and issues; building community *infrastructure* (through establishing networks, work with existing groups) to bring individuals and groups together; *organizational development* (lobbying, policy work) to encourage organizations to change in response to identified needs; and a participatory strategy aimed at involving MWHSWM in the project, particularly its decision-making processes (e.g. establishing advisory groups, involving users in steering groups). Underlying this overall strategy were important CD principles relating to working from established need, encouraging consultation and participation, and a firm commitment to equal opportunities. Above all the CD approach was about working collectively in a way that encourages a holistic view of health. For a more detailed discussion, see Miller, (1994) and Prout and Deverell (1992, 1995).

2   Our allegiance to social constructionist ideas does not mean that we see sexuality, or any other behaviour, as purely social in origin. We recognize the importance of biology and psychology. We take social construction to mean the form and meanings given to biology. Behaviour arises from a complex interaction which means that it does not really make sense analytically to try and separate out the biological and the social into distinct wholes (see Treichler, 1993).

3   A similar experience was related by Mark Kjeldsen of the London Streetwise

outreach project. He reported that when men were asked about their sexuality for the purposes of monitoring, their answers would not fall into his fixed categories but would be of the type '50% bisexual, 10% gay, 40% heterosexual.'

4   A detailed account and discussion of the policy and practice issues raised by the MESMAC project is given in Prout and Deverell (1995).

References

ALMAGUER, T. (1993) 'Chicano men: A cartography of homosexual identity and behaviour', in ABELOVE, H., BARALE, M.A. and HALPERIN, M. (Eds) *The Lesbian and Gay Studies Reader*, London: Routledge.

ALONSO, A.M., and KOPRECK, M.T. (1993) 'Silences: 'Hispanics,' AIDS, and sexual practices', in ABELOVE, H., BARALE, M.A. and HALPERIN, M. (Eds) *The Lesbian and Gay Studies Reader*, London: Routledge.

ALTMAN, D. (1988) 'Legitimation through disaster: AIDS and the gay movement', in FEE, E. and FOX, D. (Eds) *AIDS The Burdens of History*, London: University of California Press.

BARTOS, M., McLEOD, J. and NOTT, P. (1993) 'Meanings of sex between men', a study conducted by the Australian Federation of AIDS Organisations for the Commonwealth Department of Health, Housing, Local Government and Community Services, Canberra.

BOULTON, M. and WEATHERBURN, P. (1990) 'Literature review on bisexuality and HIV transmission', London, Academic Department of Public Health, St. Mary's Medical School (mimeo).

BERUBE, A and ESCOFFIER, J. (1991) 'Queer nation', *Out/Look*, Winter, 14–23.

BRAH, A. (1992) 'Difference, diversity and differentiation', in DONALD, J. and RATTANSI, A. (Eds) *'Race', Culture and Difference*, London: Sage.

BRAKE, M. (1976) 'I may be a queer, but at least I am a man: male hegemony and ascribed versus achieved gender', in BARKER, D. and ALLEN, S. (Eds) *Sexual Divisions and Society: Process and Change*, London: Tavistock.

BRITISH MARKET RESEARCH BUREAU (1992) 'Gay pubs and clubs 1992: Report on a quantitative survey', London, BMRB (mimeo).

BUTLER, J. (1993) 'Imitation and gender insubordination', in ABELOVE, H., BARALE, M.A. and HALPERIN, M. (Eds) *The Lesbian and Gay Studies Reader*, London: Routledge.

DADA, M. (1990) 'Race and the AIDS agenda', in BOFFIN, T. and GUPTA, S. (Eds) *Ecstatic Antibodies Revisiting the AIDS Mythology*, London: Rivers Oram Press.

DAVIES, P.M. (1990) 'Some problems in defining and sampling non-heterosexual males', Project SIGMA Working Paper No. 3., London, South Bank Polytechnic.

DAVIS, M.D., KLEMMER, U. and DOWSETT, G.W. (1991) *'Bisexually active men and beats: Theoretical and educational implications'*, Sydney: AIDS Council for New South Wales and 'Macquarie University AIDS Research Unit.

DEVERELL, K. (1992) 'Outreach Work in Saunas: The Experience of Leicester Black MESMAC', MESMAC Evaluation Working Paper No.4, Keele University, Department of Sociology and Social Anthropology (mimeo).

DEVERELL, K. and DOYLE, T. (1992) 'MESMAC Leeds: An Evaluation of the Establishment of a Lesbian and Gay Theatre Group', MESMAC Evaluation Working Paper No.6, Keele University, Department of Sociology and Social Anthropology (mimeo).

DEVERELL, K. and PROUT, A. (1992) 'MESMAC Tyneside: Working with Men on a Housing Estate', MESMAC Evaluation Working Paper No.1, Keele University: Department of Sociology and Social Anthropology (mimeo).

FUJIMURA, J.H. (1992) 'Crafting science: Standardised packages, boundary objects, and "Translation"', in PICKERING, A. (Ed.) *Science as Practice and Culture*, Chicago: Chicago University Press.

GATTER, P. (1991) 'On Neutral Ground? The culture of HIV/AIDS voluntary organisations in London', London, South Bank Polytechnic (mimeo).

GATTER, P. (1993) 'Anthropology and the culture of HIV/AIDS Voluntary organisations', in AGGLETON, P., DAVIES, P. and HART, G. (Eds) *AIDS: Facing the Second Decade*, London: Falmer Press.

HALL, S. (1990) 'Cultural identity and diaspora', in RUTHERFORD, J. (Ed.) *Identity Community, Culture, Difference*, London: Lawrence and Wishart.

HARAWAY, D. (1990) 'A manifesto for cyborgs: Science, technology, and socialist feminism in the 1980s', in NICHOLSON, L.J. (Ed.) *Feminism/Post modernism*, London: Routledge.

KING, E. (1993) *Safety in Numbers*, London: Cassell.

KIPPAX, S., CRAWFORD, J., CONNELL, R.W., DOWSETT, G.W., WATSON, L., RODDEN, P. *et al.* (1990) 'The Importance of Gay Community in the Prevention of HIV Transmission', Social Aspects of the Prevention of AIDS Study A, Report No.7, Sydney, Macquarie University.

MANUEL, P., FANI-KOYODE R., and GUPTA, S. (1989) 'Imaging black sexuality', in REEVES, M. and HAMMOND, J. (Eds) *Looking Beyond the Frame: Racism, Representation and Resistance*, (Links 34), Oxford: Third World First.

MARTIN, R. (1990) *Definitions of Community Work*, London: Federation of Community Work Training Groups.

MARTIN, B. (1993) 'Lesbian identity and autobiographical difference(s)', in ABELOVE, H., BARALE, M.A. and HALPERIN, D.M. (Eds) *The Lesbian and Gay Studies Reader*, London: Routledge.

MILLER, D. (1994) (Ed.) *The MESMAC Guide: A Practical Resource For Community-Based HIV Prevention With Gay and Bisexual Men and Other Men Who Have Sex With Men*, London: Health Education Authority.

MURRAY, S. (1992) 'Components of gay community in San Francisco', in HERDT, G. (Ed.) *Gay Culture in America: Essays from the Field*, Boston: Beacon Press.

PADGUG, R. (1989) 'Sexual matters: rethinking sexuality in history', in DUBERMAN, R.B., VICINUS, M. and CHAUNCEY, G. (Eds) *Hidden from History: Reclaiming the Lesbian and Gay Past*, London: Penguin.

PATTON, C. (1985) *Sex and Germs – The Politics of AIDS*, Boston: South End Press.

PATTON, C. (1990) *Inventing AIDS*, London: Routledge.

PETERSON, J.L. (1992) 'Black men and their same-sex desires and behaviors', in HERDT, G. (Ed.) *Gay Culture in America: Essays from the Field*, Boston: Beacon Press.

PLUMMER, K. (1975) *Sexual stigma: an interactive account*, London: Routledge and Kegan Paul.

PRESTAGE, G. and HOOD, D. (1993) 'Targetting non-gay attached men who have sex with men: New data, outreach and cultural issues', paper given at the Seventh Social Aspects of AIDS Conference, London.

PROUT, A. and DEVERELL K. (1992) 'The Impact of the MESMAC project:an interim review', MESMAC Evaluation Working Paper No.5, Keele University, Department of Sociology and Social Anthropology (mimeo).

PROUT, A. and DEVERELL, K. (1995) *Working with Diversity-Building Communities: Evaluating the Mesmac Project*, London: Health Education Authority.

RUST, P.C. (1993) '"Coming out" in the age of social constructionism: Sexual identity formation among lesbian and bisexual women', *Gender and Society*, **7**(1), 50–77.

RUTHERFORD, J.(1990) 'A place called home: Identity and the cultural politics of difference', in RUTHERFORD, J. (Ed.) *Identity Community, Culture, Difference*, London: Lawrence and Wishart.

SCOTT, P. (1993) 'Beginning HIV prevention work with gay and bisexual men', in EVANS, B., SANDBERG, S. and WATSON, S. (Eds.) *Healthy Alliances in HIV Prevention*, London: Health Education Authority.

SHEFFIELD HEALTH AUTHORITY (1993) *Community Development and Health: The Way Forward in Sheffield*, Sheffield: Healthy Sheffield Support Team.

SIEGAL, K. and BAUMAN, L. (1986) 'Methodological issues in AIDS-related research', in FELDMAN, D. and JOHNSON, T. (Eds) *The Social Dimensions of AIDS, Method and Theory*, London: Praeger.

SMITHIES, J. (1991) 'Organisation and community development', unpublished thesis, Sheffield Business School.

STAR, S.L. and GRIESMER, J.R. (1989) 'Institutional ecology, translations and boundary objects: Amateurs and professionals in Berkeley's Museum of Vertebrate Zoology', 1907–39', *Social Studies of Science*, **19**, 387–420.

TREICHLER, P.A., (1993) 'AIDS, HIV and the cultural construction of reality', in HERDT, G. and LINDENBAUM, S. (Eds) *The Time of AIDS: Social Analysis, Theory and Method*, London: Sage.

VANCE, C. (1989) 'Social construction theory: Problems in the history of sexuality', in ALTMAN, D. *et al.* (Eds) *Homosexuality, Which Homosexuality?*, London: Gay Men's Press.

VANCE, C. (1991) 'Anthropology rediscovers sexuality: A theoretical comment', *Social Science Medicine*, **33**(8), 875–84.

WATNEY, S. (1993) 'Emergent sexual identities and HIV/AIDS', in AGGLETON, P., DAVIES, P. and HART, G. (Eds) *AIDS: Facing the Second Decade*, London: Taylor and Francis.

WEATHERBURN, P., *et al.* (1992) *The Sexual Lifestyles of Gay and Bisexual Men in England and Wales*, London: Department of Health.

WEEKS, J. (1986) *Sexuality*, London: Tavistock.

WEEKS, J. (1989) 'AIDS, altruism, and the new right', in CARTER, E. and WATNEY, S. (Eds) *Taking Liberties AIDS and Cultural Politics*, London: Serpent's Tail.

WEEKS, J. (1990) 'The Value of Difference', in RUTHERFORD, J. (Ed.) *Identity, Community, Culture, Difference*, London: Lawrence and Wishart.

Chapter 13

Discourses of Power and Empowerment in the Fight Against HIV/AIDS in Africa

Carolyn Baylies and Janet Bujra

AIDS in Africa is transmitted largely through heterosexual sex in a context of gender inequality. Controlling the AIDS epidemic therefore requires a transformation in gender relations as much as it requires miracle cures or technological 'fixes'. In this situation the 'empowerment' of women has often been advocated as a strategy and a solution. In practice, transformations in gender relations are hard-won against the embedded structures of male power, even where, as in the case of AIDS, sexual relations put men at risk too. If the reality of power is neglected, the call for empowerment may remain little more than a slogan.

In devising a research project on the significance of gender relations to addressing the AIDS epidemic in Tanzania and Zambia we became aware of a paradox.[1] On the one hand, in the literature of development studies and practical activism, the concept of empowerment was, and is, much in favour. Empowerment is offered as a form of strategic intervention aimed at harnessing the creative energies of those who might previously have been seen as 'victims' ('women', 'communities', 'the poor'). In this literature, however, it is rare for either the concept of empowerment, or that of power – which it clearly entails – to be theorized.

Conversely, in the sociological literature, where theories of power (and thereby implicitly, theories of empowerment) used to be central, post-structuralist and postmodernist thought has questioned the very concept of power, rendering it indeterminate and pluralistic, and the social categories that it reified, such as 'men', or 'the working class' as essentialist or universalistic, and in need of deconstruction. Some feminists were adopting the language of postmodernism in a way that appeared to us potentially disempowering – perhaps not in the academic sphere, but certainly in the life and death field of AIDS research and action.

Feminism is relevant to our research as our focus is on the means by which women in general might be enabled to protect themselves and their families from the threat of HIV/AIDS, and on the difficulties they may encounter in the process. It aims to build on the pioneering work of Schoepf (1991), Ankrah (1991), Ulin (1992), Obbo (1993) and others. Focusing on women in particular will allow us to investigate the ways, both individual and collective, in which women can protect themselves against the threat of HIV/AIDS. It does not assume that women are a homogeneous category, but that women's already accumulated experience of organizing and networking in their varying social locations may be adaptable to the struggle against HIV/AIDS.

HIV/AIDS work in Africa demands that we look critically, though not dismissively, at the concept of empowerment – as theory, methodology and as a strategy for change. This assessment propels us to ask how and why theories of power were lost to social analysis and whether they need to be revived. We will make a preliminary attempt to do this through a review of literature in which the concept of empowerment figures, with the aim of identifying common themes and problems. The literature in question spans a wide range of interdisciplinary fields.

Power, Disempowerment and Empowerment

An example drawn from the work of Brooke Schoepf and her colleagues in Zaire (Schoepf *et al.*, 1991) both highlights the way in which AIDS raises issues of gendered power and underlines the inseparability of gender from other social relations of inequality. It reveals how the questioning of the efficacy of condoms in the media served to undermine the resolve of sex workers to confront their clients with new terms designed to enhance mutual protection.

In 1988, a US 'sex researcher' was quoted by *Paris Match* as saying that condoms provide incomplete protection from HIV infection. While not inaccurate, the comment was unhelpful given the absence of any totally effective form of prevention other than abstinence. *Paris Match* circulates not just in France but around the French-speaking world, and in Zaire it was read by the small élite of better-off and educated people, among them male university students, some of whom visited prostitutes in poor areas of Kinshasa. At a time when these women were trying to put into effect a programme to ensure that their clients wore condoms, they were told by the relatively high-status students that there was 'no need to use those things', on the grounds that it had now been 'proved' that condoms were useless (Schoepf *et al.*, 1991: p. 198). The women needed to work to provide for themselves and their children. Having had little formal education, they were also largely illiterate as well as poor. They believed the students. Their determination diminished and condom use decreased.

Knowledge from some sources has more potency than knowledge from others, and this potency is socially defined through asymmetrical relations of class, neo-colonialism and gender. In this case its authority was lent by 'science', communicated by a magazine published in the north (as against local public campaign advocating condom use), and relayed by 'educated' locals (and by men as opposed to women). Women, literally at the bottom of this hierarchy, could not sustain their own painfully acquired views.

If this were the whole story, then prospects would be dire indeed. But women do have the capacity to resist male power in certain circumstances. Examples from Africa illustrate the potential, through collective action, for women to link private concerns (in this case the fear of infection within sexual relations) to the public domain. Theorizing these actions is more problematic, but crucial to promoting the empowerment of women as a strategy.

Feminism and the Theorisation of Power/Empowerment

In the context of gender-aware campaigns against HIV/AIDS in the 1990s, a feminist slogan of the 1960s, 'the personal is political' could easily assume new significance. Sadly, feminism has since taken a depoliticizing turn – at least in Europe and America. Along with this, its forceful analysis of the structural basis of gendered power relations has been muted.

New-wave feminism provided a most successful prototype for movements of empowerment in the way it spread through networking and consciousness-raising groups. The consciousness raising group was eminently fitted to the philosophy of new-wave feminism in its voluntaristic, non-hierarchical organizational form and in its role as a venue within which women could share private concerns in a way that rendered them public and political. Despite its contradictions (Coote and Campbell, 1987; Freeman, 1971), the consciousness-raising group worked to empower many women. Its philosophy and tactics owed more to radical feminism than to any other form of women's liberation.

It is impossible to do justice to the range of feminist writing on the question of power, since this would entail a review of the whole of new-wave feminism in its various forms (radical, liberal, Marxist/socialist, etc), all in their various ways founded on a critique of male power and an exposure of the practice of male domination. Radical feminism was the most forthright, if also the most reductionist in its earliest formulations (notably Firestone's declaration that, 'the sexual imbalance of power is biologically based', 1970: 10). Whilst deeply flawed, it could be argued that the short-term revolutionary impact of this position was related to its essentialist conception of masculinity, with men seen unequivocally as 'the enemy'.

Liberal feminists adopted a classic individualistic approach to power in which free and equal individuals had natural rights to choices and opportunities and where politics was conceived as a pluralistic and competitive process. From Wollstonecraft onwards, their challenge was to the gendered nature of the archetypal individual. What men could achieve so too could women. A woman, said Betty Friedan, must 'compete impersonally in society, as men do', she must take part in decision making, 'not as a "housewife", but as a "citizen"' (1963: 360).

Marxist and socialist feminists have been accused of harbouring a 'desire to ... exempt men from responsibility for the oppression of women' (Delphy, 1980: 104) and for attempting to foist onto feminism an ungendered conception of power founded on the class relations of production and their expression in state domination. That the power of men is very often tied in with their organized class/political power is one of the strengths of this position; but the potential for an orthodox marxist approach to render gender invisible is a serious liability.

Various formulations have attempted to harness marxist methodology to an appreciation of the importance of gender or to plant gender within a marxist position on class. These have included dualistic conceptions where class and gender are animated within separate systems, the argument that gender is ideologically encoded in class relations, or the claim that experiential knowledge renders them inseparable (for a discussion see Barrett, 1980). Addressing the role of the Senegalese state *vis à vis* multinational companies and local private capital in the transformation of gendered relations of horticulture, for example, Mackintosh insists that gender relations are 'integral to the way classes are structured and reproduced – and experienced' (1989: 37). Neither, she suggests, is reducible to or fully determined by the other.

In our view this approach continues to have considerable weight. If it complicates the research process, it also demands an appreciation of the complexity of those interacting factors that influence consciousness and action, that both define lines of conflict and facilitate collective action. Not just gender and class, but the intricacies of ethnicity and culture need to be taken into account, further magnifying but also enriching the research endeavour.[2] Despite its strengths, this stance has been eclipsed in recent years by the rise of postmodernism.

At the same time that development studies were discovering gender issues and the notion of empowerment was infiltrating the development literature as a broader strategy for dealing with development issues (see below), feminism was questioning its earlier certainties. Paradoxically, its own language of liberation, and its revaluing of experience as a source of women's strength and knowledge was increasingly turned inwards in a divisive period of fragmentation and conflict around 'identity politics'. Differences between women –

theoretical and political as well as social – came to the fore and began to be construed through intellectual engagement with poststructuralist and post-modernist thought. The appropriation and adoption by some feminists of conceptual language that seemed aptly to describe their predicament also soon became evident, with the increasing use of terms such as difference, plurality, deconstruction, etc. The depoliticizing impact of this was recognized early: 'the postmodernist point of view is explicitly hostile to any political project beyond the ephemeral' (Barrett, 1987:34; and later Mohanty, 1992; Ramazanoglu, 1993).

In this chapter our concern is not to explore the now extensive debates between feminism and postmodernism (see e.g. Barrett and Phillips, 1992; Lovibond, 1990; Ramazanoglu, 1993 and many others), but to assess the impact of postmodernism on feminist understandings of power and empower-ment, and to appreciate the significance of this for the struggle against HIV/AIDS. For the irony is, that despite a recognition of the depoliticizing sting in the tail of postmodernism, 'power' is seen to be one of the concerns that it has addressed in a novel way. Here the key engagement seems to have been with Michel Foucault (see e.g. Delsing, 1991; Gatens, 1992; McNeil, 1993; Ramaza-noglu, 1993).

As with other postmodernist writers, Foucault's thought exemplifies the break with Enlightenment philosophies of reason and progress and with the metanarrative or totalizing (and largely structuralist) theories that were built on them. There are three aspects of Foucault's work that seem to have caught the imagination of feminists, and which appear relevant to our concerns here. The first is his distinction between the power of the state and processes of power/discipline in daily life. The second lies in the understanding of power as discursive; while the third is evidenced in his work on the body and sexuality.

The distinction in Foucault's early work between power embodied in state sovereignty, and power as discipline/surveillance in everyday life is an important one, with the latter manifested in 'the gaze' and in discourses of normalization (1979, 1980a). The thesis has appeared seductive to many feminists, even as some attempted to adapt it subversively to incorporate gender (e.g. Barrett, 1991; Pringle and Watson, 1992). However, Foucault's turning away from a structural conception of society in which the state is dominant for one characterized by 'a multiform production of relations of domination' (1980b: 142), not only obviates any need to critically analyse how and why state power has so often excluded and marginalized women, but it also deprives the process of empowerment of any focus. When AIDS activists in Zambia address 'an open letter to policy makers' as well as to 'ordinary citizens' it is because only the state has the resources to effectively confront the AIDS epidemic (Weekly Post, 21 January 1994).

The second aspect is exemplified in the later work of Foucault. Here power is characterized as impersonal and pervasive, embodied in competing and diverse discourses (Foucault, 1984). Politics is redefined as discursive struggles. Ramazanoglu (1993: 24) insists that:

> From Foucault's perspective it does not make sense to think of political change, as feminists have conventionally done, in terms of emancipation from oppression. It does make sense to think of transforming political relations through the production of new discourses and so new forms of power and new forms of self.

Ramazanoglu is sceptical, arguing that male domination 'cannot be seen simply as a product of discourse, because it must also be understood as 'extra-discursive' or relating to wider realities than those of discourse' (Ramazanoglu, 1993: 22). Inevitably, this brings back into focus those 'structures' and structured processes whose understanding is attempted in theories which postmodernism has rejected. While discursive struggles may well deserve close attention, neglect of the underlying structures that inform and shape them may result in only partial understanding, rendering analysis inadequate and any practice following from it potentially self-defeating.

The third and linked aspect of Foucault's work that might seem particularly pertinent to the issue of HIV/AIDS is that which centres on the body, and on the politics of the body. Yet, as many feminists have noted, the body in question is male, and feminists had already been working on the same idea (though as Bordo perceptively remarks, they saw themselves not as developing 'a new intellectual paradigm' but as 'participating in a political movement' (Bordo, 1993: 181). Adapting Foucault's frame to female bodies has produced some fascinating excursions on the subject of the body as produced and disciplined, and the body as a site for creative and subversive self-determination. While this illuminates the social and historical shaping of the individual human form, it throws little light on the question of the relationship of bodies in sexual encounters. Indeed, Foucault perceived his work on sexuality as an analysis of 'the modality of relation to the self', or discourses of personal morality in relation to sex, rather than sexual relations themselves (in Rabinow, 1984: 338).[3]

Borrowing from Foucault it can be conceded that the operation of power is illuminated by consideration of discursive practices. Although not necessarily adopting Foucault's conceptual language, the literature on AIDS reveals an appreciation of this general point through its discussion of 'representational images', 'beliefs', 'health education messages', 'ideology', 'sexual terminology', etc. One example is the way in which the presentation of AIDS in the media is both gendered and racialized; another is the use of sexual terminology in health education in Uganda (see, for example, Kitzinger and Miller, 1991; Pitts and Jackson, 1993; Ssali *et al.*, 1992). One particularly fine and nuanced example of the use of Foucauldian discourse analysis in relation to Africa is found in Seidel (1993) where attention is paid to competing discourses of HIV/AIDS: discourses of 'rights' and of 'empowerment' as well as those of 'control' and 'exclusion'. Medical discourse (that which has the most potency in the field at present) could well be usefully subjected to Foucault's (1980c: 118) characterization as a discourse that produces 'effects of truth'.

One current controversy regarding the relationship between HIV and AIDS in Africa (whipped up into a bitter scientific debate by *The Sunday Times*) could be regarded through the same lens, though the competing views here both operate within Enlightenment parameters, with the assumption that the application of reason and positivistic method will lead to the resolution of problems: the search for a definition, an epidemiology, and a cure for AIDS. The language is that of 'truth'. As a recent headline in *New Scientist* put it, the link between HIV and AIDS is 'beyond reasonable doubt' (15 January 1994) whilst AIDS activists in Zambia rebut the argument with 'the hard facts' of deaths and the dying (*Weekly Post,* 'An open letter to policy makers and ordinary citizens', 21 January 1994). It is important to recall, however, that discursive 'effects' borrow force from the social position of those who employ them (as illustrated by the Zairean example above).

One of the more sympathetic attempts to apply Foucauldian insights to the question of sexuality in the era of AIDS nevertheless concludes that women's vulnerability to male power is not explicable 'wholly in terms of discourses of sexuality, or power situated in the intimate relationships of sexual encounters' and that 'Foucault's notion of resistance is very different from feminist notions of women's empowerment because his definition of power underestimates the intransigence of the powerful in defending their privilege . . .' (Ramazanoglu and Holland, 1993: 260, 254).

Women's concern to protect themselves still has to confront the real power of men over women's bodies and minds – the pimp with the knife, the violent husband, the husband with customary law on his side, the male client on whom a woman depends for a livelihood, the loving husband who refuses to use condoms. It also has to challenge other sources of power that men exercise over each other: economic, political and legal, and which in Africa force some men to travel long distances in search of work, deprive others of land or leave them in extreme poverty – all factors conducive to the spread of life-threatening disease. These factors are not products of discourse, though the way we talk about them undoubtedly is. To aim to understand or confront them simply in terms of discourse analysis is to operate with one hand tied behind our backs.

It is not that we advocate a simple return to the comforting formulas of the metanarrative, the grand theory which could 'explain all'. Limitations of the various theoretical positions on power devised prior to the postmodernist onslaught must be acknowledged. Gatens reconsiders some of these (especially liberal and Marxist versions) and exposes their inadequacies, though she says little of their strengths (1992). Davis, Leijenaar and Oldersma (1991) address more 'conventional' sociological theories of power along with Foucault – e.g. Lukes, Giddens and Gramsci – and find some mileage in doing this. There is little value in abandoning ourselves to postmodernism when other theoretical approaches – those which recognize structural constraints as well as others which illuminate power relations through interactional analysis – seem more serviceable both to feminism and in the context of women's struggles against the threat of HIV/AIDS. Conversely, such insights as may emerge from a postmodernist approach and which would deepen our understanding of gendered power relations and the potential for resistance and transformation should be acknowledged.

Development Theory and HIV/AIDS

Schuurman (1993) and others have described a current impasse in development theory which is partly attributable to a postmodernist critique paralleling that which has confronted feminism. At the same time, Schuurman argues, feminism has exerted an independent contribution to this impasse through its insistent exposure of the 'invisibility of women' in the mainstream discourse on development (Schuurman, 1993: 32). In his view, the paralysis in development theory has been variously marked either by political nihilism or by a Utopian faith in the liberatory and empowering rise of 'new social movements'.

Development studies has been particularly marked by an Enlightenment belief in social improvement. It has also been characterized by the use of structural frameworks of analysis. The issue of power was a key one, although in its various theoretical formulations it was perceived to inhere in a variety of subjects. In the 1960s, modernization theorists, such as Lerner (1964), used to argue that traditional forms of authoritarian government were a barrier to economic development, and that 'participatory lifeways' would enhance the innovatory spirit in society and facilitate the thrusting achievement of 'new men'. In rejecting this perspective, dependency theory delineated power as residing in metropolitan control of the capitalist world market and in the centripetal flow of 'surplus'. Against this force, third-world states could exhibit limited leverage. Marxist critiques of dependency theory focused on the state and on exploitative class relations, both on the local and on the international level, as a primary source of limited economic growth.

The capacity of these various perspectives to account for an increasing divergence of experience, with a vibrant economic advance in some regions and stagnation and increasing indebtedness in others, coupled with world economic recession and the collapse of Eastern European socialist regimes, led to a questioning of their explanatory value. And yet an important thread of continuity may be discerned in that perspective which has characteristically underlain the activities of the international financial institutions (IFIs) and come to exert a hegemonic influence on the contours of third world development. Echoes of the earlier modernization approach resonate strongly in what has been referred to as new right theory or neo-liberalism, which applauds the free reign of market forces (at least for the developing world) and celebrates 'democracy' and 'good governance'. Ostensibly appearing more in tune with the decentred view of the world proposed by postmodernist thought, there is probably a greater hegemonic impact of the current dominant discourse in the area of development (under the aegis of the International Monetary Fund/World Bank) than has occurred previously. Yet, as a further irony, these same dominant actors (which are increasingly dictating a uniform set of economic policies) have also adopted a rhetoric of participation, which if taken to its logical conclusion might yield disparate and innovative approaches. Thus, while projecting a philosophy based on the satisfaction of human needs, participation, democracy, sustainable development, the enhancement of welfare and the eradication of poverty, the IFIs have managed global indebtedness and imposed economic and political policies on weakened third-world states that have not only exacerbated poverty and welfare deficits but have also led to some very cynical formulas for 'democratic' government.

There is a sense in which the AIDS epidemic stands as a metaphor for the impasse in development theory and the limitations of IFI initiatives. First, it poses quite new and disturbing issues that turn conventional thinking on its head. Population growth with its impact on the environment and on society and economy has often been taken to be a key problem (sometimes *the* key problem) in developing countries (e.g. World Bank, 1990). The global epidemic of AIDS suggests the need for fundamental reconsideration of this perspective, particularly in the case of Africa. The prospect is now one of a reduced rate of population growth, but more significantly, the decimation of the 'youngest and fittest' – those in their prime productive and reproductive years – with its attendant threat to the sustainability of peasant agriculture as well as all other economic and social activities. Women find themselves at the sharp end of this problem, as it is on them that ultimately the burden falls of reproductive decision-making in the context of sexual relations, which now carry potentially fatal consequences both for women and their unborn children. All are at risk, and yet women are the most powerless to resist.

Secondly, the role of the state in responding to this crisis has been undermined everywhere in Africa by structural adjustment policies that demand a contraction in state subsidies for the health, education and welfare of their peoples, and from which the immiseration of the population follows almost inexorably. In Zambia, for example, now that medicines are no longer 'free' at the point of need, people with AIDS are prescribed medication, that they cannot afford to buy, to alleviate their symptoms. The weakness of states in Africa to resist pressure to liberalize and adjust is exposed at the very time that they need to be strong. The 'social marketing' of condoms, subsidized by USAID, is one example of the forceful opening up of the market. Social marketing is a 'success story' in terms of the new economic philosophy: condoms are sold through outlets such as bars and markets 'like Coca Cola'.[4] But the supply is controlled by American interests using a local partner, preferably from the private sector. As Winsbury (1992) notes, the new process: 'bypasses entirely the conventional state channels of procurement and distribution ... so further emphasising the private enterprise approach to the condom'. The need for continuing analysis of the diverse linkages between global power, local states and the class relations of capitalist production is evident, at the same time as new and practical strategies are required to confront the issue.

Development Practice: Issues of Participation and Empowerment

One of the key strategies here has been empowerment. While appropriated as little more than virtuous rhetoric by some actors on the international scene, it also figures in the emergence of methodological tools devised by development practitioners over the last decade and a half which are genuinely attuned to a recasting of hierarchy. Such methodologies, encompassing research, planning and project implementation, represent attempts to make development practice work better by being more responsive to the circumstances of local people – the 'beneficiaries' of development efforts. The aim has been to ensure that development interventions will be acceptable to them and can be easily incorporated into their 'world' – into the existing division of labour and into the time and space dimensions of recipient communities.

Yet the focus has not always been actual empowerment, so much as lubrication of the implementation process, with a pragmatic view to ensuring that the efforts and funds of external agents are not wasted. This is illustrated in an account by Salmen (1987) who was commissioned by the World Bank to live with project beneficiaries in the low-income areas of two Latin American cities in order to gain an understanding of the development projects from the participants' point of view. The manual he produced describes a methodology – participant observation evaluation – intended to ensure greater understanding of who beneficiaries are and what they want, and to facilitate the maintenance of communication with them so as to highlight any difficulties that may arise from misunderstandings or inadequate knowledge during the process of project implementation.

Salmen describes this methodological intervention as providing project managers with better intelligence so that they can do their jobs more effectively. It does not empower beneficiaries but rather facilitates the rational exercise of power by those at the 'top' (including national or international development agencies such as the World Bank). Long and Villareal (1993: 160) have identified this as 'the managerialist and interventionist undertones inherent in development work'. A different emphasis, and one which bears more directly on empowerment, is evidenced in the call for beneficiaries to directly participate in project planning and research, rather than simply being 'voices' assisting project management. A number of such participatory methodologies, variously linked to direct action, or making explicit claims about the relationship between participation and power, have emerged in recent years in the development project field – among them 'participatory social research', 'participatory action research' and 'participatory rural appraisal'.

An early contribution by Indian scholars/developmentalists (Fernandes and Tandon, 1981) argued that participatory social research and action should entail the abandonment of hierarchical distributions of power between researchers and so-called subjects, and substitute a 'horizontal distribution'. Participatory social action should involve beneficiaries themselves becoming agents of social action and thereby reduce power differentials between those who control and those who need resources.

Similar principles underlie participatory action research, whose advocates have referred to a democratization of the research process and shared ownership, both of this process and its outcome, and to stimulating community action 'by instilling among participants a sense of immediacy and personal identification with the discovery process' (Maclure and Bassey, 1991). Participatory action research is described as involving a partnership, whereby decision making and control are shared by all those having a stake in the outcome. Ideally it involves community-based learning, whereby participating groups are enabled to analyse their own situations and attempt to devise solutions.

Advocates of a related methodology, participatory rural appraisal, suggest that the role of the expert outsider is not to collect data, but to facilitate local people in assessing their own knowledge. This approach evolved in relation to agricultural projects, where, according to Chambers (1992), the challenge is not to improve the professional's analysis, but to help farmers 'do their own analysis and to do it better'. Edwards (1993) argues that such methods 'facilitate joint action among agencies and the people with whom they are working, to enable them to *understand social structure and development issues* within a given location' (our emphasis: 89).

Whilst participatory methods are now, in Edwards' view 'almost taken for granted in development work' (Edwards, 1993: 89), they are not without their critics. Participation can be an empty slogan, or be very limited in its practical implementation. A purist would argue that it should apply at all stages – the definition of needs, the design of the project, the process of research, the implementation of a project, its evaluation, maintenance, or utilization of the knowledge gained. In practice this is rarely achieved and participation seldom extends beyond the middle stages.

Some of the issues raised can be illustrated from the HIV/AIDS field. Seeley *et al.* (1992) in an analysis of community based participatory research in Uganda, note some 'unsolved problems'. The central one is the way that, in the health field, 'communities' are often treated as undifferentiated, devoid of internal power relations or divergent interests. Seeley *et al.* note that it was those already well-placed in the local political structures who came forward to take part in the project's work, and that locally employed staff were regarded by others as 'growing fat' at the expense of the rest of the community. They also note the folly of overlooking differences along the lines of religion or ethnicity, and the way in which people's anxiety and fears about infection isolate them rather than augmenting community solidarity. In relation to HIV/AIDS, medical personnel are also unlikely to seek out villagers as the source of 'knowledge'. (As Rahnema perceptively remarks, 'no-one learns who claims to know already in advance' (1992: 122)). Given that the project carried out by Seeley *et al.*, like many others, was externally funded (by the British Government), it is hardly surprising that the design was also externally imposed: 'it has been for the community, after accepting the presence of the Programme in the area, to look for ways to benefit from its presence' (Seeley *et al.*, 1992: 1095).

There is clearly a link between participatory methodologies and feminist questioning of positivist research methods. Though feminists may have asked more searching questions about practice (Opie, 1992), affirmation of the need to question power relations operating in the research process, seeking to ensure ownership of the process of research by its subjects and democratizing research have a strong resonance in the literature on feminist methodology. Parallels can also be drawn with emancipatory methodology developed by researchers in the field of disability or with interactionist models of power and decision making developed in some schools of sociology and critically applied to the development field by writers such as Long (1990).

Where participation has been seen as the appropriate process, empowerment is often understood as its product, both as an end in itself and as a means towards achieving larger social goals. The notion of empowerment in the literature is not always used consistently or rigorously, or always associated with a clear theoretical understanding of what power is or how it is exercised. Nor does an invoking of empowerment as a virtue always imply a careful theorizing of either its feasibility or its implications for existing power relations. The call for empowerment logically assumes that some sections of the population are disadvantaged and powerless, and that there is a link between their lack of power and their material disadvantage (or, in the case of AIDS, their vulnerability to infection). It implies the existence of power relations, an asymmetry of power, though it does not usually identify the theoretical origin of this power – for example, as founded in the 'deep structures' of society (e.g. production relations), or as constructed through negotiation, or identifiable only at the level of discourse.

Where power is conceded, the call for empowerment appears magically to dissolve it. As one of its most fervent advocates argues, the approach is 'centred on people and their environment rather than production and profits', and whilst this form of alternative development from below 'cannot be "guided" by governing elites' it 'requires a strong state … an agile and responsive state, accountable to its citizens' (Friedmann, 1992: 31, 33, 35). Large claims can then be made for its efficacy: 'If poverty is a condition of relative disempowerment … then a key to the overcoming of mass poverty is the social and political empowerment of the poor' (Friedmann, 1992: viii). The irony inherent in the image of a strong state somehow distanced from production and profits and oriented toward protecting the poor and dis-advantaged as against those economically privileged should not escape comment. Formulations such as that of Friedmann beg a theory of the state which links power relations within civil society to those embodied in the state.

If empowerment approaches have been taken up by those on the libertarian left (and could be said to contain a good deal of wishful thinking), they have also seemed expedient to those more to the right. As one of us has remarked elsewhere: 'the promise of liberation in the concept of empower-ment is blunted by its uneasy coexistence with other shibboleths of current [official] development discourse, especially "cost-effectiveness" [and] "sus-tainability", and with the demands of political conditionality that development be "democratic" or "participatory"' (Bujra, 1993: 69). The call for empower-ment can become a device for gaining the consent of 'beneficiaries,' their 'ownership' of a project being a means for ensuring its maintenance. In this sense it verges on an opportunistic exploitation of the poor. It is noteworthy that the social categories targeted for empowerment initiatives are relatively unthreatening – 'the poor' or 'rural communities' for example. Empowering wage labourers is rarely on the agenda.

Empowerment approaches can also transfer the responsibility for trans-formation from the powerful to those who are most disadvantaged and lacking in resources. And who more disadvantaged than women? In an article on women's access to health care in developing countries it is argued that: 'Women must become agents of change to improve their situation … Women are seeking empowerment throughout the world' (Ojanuga and Gilbert, 1992: 616). The contradictions inherent in the word 'must' should be noted.

Empowerment in Gender Planning and Gender Aware Development

Women have never been absent as objects of development planning, but it was only when they began to speak for themselves in the 1970s and 1980s that official discourse recognized their active existence (Moser, 1993). Now lip service is paid to women's involvement in the development effort; in the World Bank and among UN and other international agencies, women have become 'the answer to everything' (Townsend, 1993: 172) and every development project has a women's component. The way in which gender has become incorporated and institutionalized is largely through a variant of liberal feminism, the Women in Development (WID) approach. For some women, gender planning must mean more than this (Young, 1993), and specifically it entails empowering women. The advocacy of empowerment recognizes that women (or some women) are specifically disadvantaged – usually relative to men, though their disadvantage may be embodied in broader legal or economic structures.

The work of two of those who have elaborated themes of empowerment, Caroline Moser (1993) and Sara Longwe (1991), can be viewed more fully as examples of this approach. If not always explicitly drawn, each contains an implicit suggestion of power being ultimately located in social structures. Moser has written extensively on the notion of gender planning, which she says 'is not an end in itself but a means by which women through a process of empowerment can emancipate themselves' (1993: 190). It operates through negotiated debate about the redistribution of power and resources at various levels – the household, society and the state. Rejecting past forms of planning that operate 'top-down' via dominant structures of power and control, she argues that change – transformative change – can only be achieved through 'bottom-up' mobilization of agency in civil society. In a key passage she writes: 'If the success of gender planning depends on the participation of women, then it is the organisation of women within civil society that requires examination' (Moser, 1993: 191).

Much of Moser's work has built upon the contrast between concepts of 'practical' and 'strategic' gender needs, originally formulated by Molyneux (1985). Practical gender needs are those that emerge from an existing gender division of labour and set of gender norms. It may be women's task to collect water. If the difficulty of obtaining water can be relieved by an intervention, such as installation of a well and pump in a village, then some of the burden of women's everyday lives will have been removed: practical gender needs will have been addressed. Strategic gender needs relate to the effects of the asymmetry of gender relations and their satisfaction is in a transformative direction, precisely because they address and attempt to alter prevailing gender relations. Training in skills otherwise restricted to men, or community provision of childcare, which removes (in part) the assumption that child care is inherently a mother's responsibility, may constitute interventions towards satisfying strategic gender needs, though more confrontational challenges to men's power may also play a part.

Satisfaction of both practical and strategic gender needs may empower. The meeting of practical gender needs, while reinforcing the existing gender division of labour, may relieve women of some burdens (drudgery) and thereby permit their engaging in other activities (e.g. literacy training), which can be seen as empowering. The meeting of strategic gender needs is more intimately bound up with empowerment in the sense of contributing to a change in the gender division of labour and in confronting the entrenched power of men.[5] Gender planning, which is sensitive to the constraints upon women and the impact of particular interventions, adds an important dimension to women's participation, enabling a more rigorous appraisal of the objectives of such participation.

Longwe has also written of the need to insert an explicit gender element in development planning. According to her, '. . . the central issue of women's development is women's empowerment, to enable women to take an equal place with men, and to participate equally in the development process . . .' (Longwe, 1991: 150). She advocates gender awareness, which for her implies a recognition that women have different needs from men. Gender-aware development initiatives, for Longwe, should seek equality and empowerment along a number of dimensions – not just improved welfare, or access to resources, or heightened consciousness, but also shared control over decision making and over present and future resources.

Avoiding the pitfalls of a Utopian sketch of what *might* or *ought* to be, is as serious a problem in some of this work as in the broader literature on participation in development. Pearson (1993) has queried the assumption that empowerment can be delivered. In pointing up the distinction between the WID approach, which in her view tends to 'add women on' to development initiatives while locating them primarily in terms of their reproductive role, and a Gender and Development (GAD) approach, which looks critically at the broad basis of gender relations, linking them both with underlying economic structures and cultural specificities, she suggests that empowerment within a WID approach is a misnomer. Whilst interventions (by NGOs and other agencies) may facilitate women in income generation or ease their work load, and may thereby promote solidarity, this does not of itself constitute empowerment, because it does not confront the inequalities of gender relations.

It is the level of *organization* amongst women that Pearson (1993) sees as the ultimate key to empowerment. A GAD approach, which she identifies with a feminist perspective, involves both consciousness and action, the collective involvement of women, organizing on the basis of their understanding of gender-based oppression. A similar argument has been put forward by Young

(1993) who stresses that while collective empowerment of women brings with it individual empowerment, it entails far more than the individual advancement which follows from those income generating activities so frequently (and misleadingly) promoted under the cloak of empowerment. Harmonizing this position with that of Moser and Longwe might entail regarding empowerment as a cumulative process, one which may initially germinate from interventions to satisfy practical problems and welfare needs, but can only be fully claimed via organization, involvement and participation imbued with consciousness of the structure/patterns of gender relations that constrain women. But it would also have to find ways of dealing with the inequalities amongst women themselves.

The emergence of AIDS raises issues both at the level of practical and strategic gender needs. Moreover, strategies of protection and prevention have frequently prioritized empowerment to counter what is construed as a situation of vulnerability and subordination for women.

Empowerment as a Strategy of Protection in the Context of HIV/AIDS

In a document commissioning research in the field of AIDS in developing countries, the British Overseas Development Administration called for work that would facilitate the 'empowerment of women to increase their capacity to protect themselves from HIV and other STDs' (2 August 1991). The World Bank, in its 1993 *World Development Report: Investing in Health,* sees AIDS as a serious threat to economic development, but still is working within the discredited model of 'high risk groups' (Holland *et al.*, 1990). Again a key solution is empowerment: 'It is important not simply to provide information on condoms but also to ensure their availability and to empower members of the core group, especially female sex workers, to use them' (World Bank, 1990: 101). It should be noted that they were not talking about female condoms here, and that no recognition of the problems women face in insisting that men use them is shown!

In the real world those affected or threatened have not waited to be empowered: they have empowered themselves. The struggle against HIV/AIDS has seen parallel movements of mobilization and initiatives of protection involving collective action in various parts of the world. It was the gay community in America that first began to see this disease as requiring a collective response. They organized themselves not only to care for and support those infected, but also to protect those still free of infection by making a link between knowledge of the forms of transmission and the need to change sexual behaviour. Organizations such as the Terrence Higgins Trust in Britain had a similar origin. They were remarkably successful in effecting changes in sexual behaviour amongst gay men, such as encouraging the practice of safer sex, and devising new norms for relating to each other – though it has been said that the impact of this has declined over time. To some extent, then, the social response to AIDS has been to stimulate voluntary action and to generate innovative forms of collective self-help – ways in which the victims themselves can support each other which have become models for work in other situations. One reason why gay men in the north were able to do this so effectively was that, as a stigmatized minority on the one hand, but a relatively affluent white middle class one on the other, they already had developed networks of support – and in some parts of America had created whole self-servicing communities (Kippax, 1992; McKevitt, 1993).

In Africa, although both men and women are affected, women are especially vulnerable. There is the tendency to see them primarily as transmitters of the virus to men or to their children ('dangerous vectors and contaminated vessels bearing condemned babies' as one source puts it: Bassett and Mhloyi, 1991: 146). There is also the tendency to place disproportionate blame on women, and especially on those who sell sexual services in order to survive. Here, both men in general and state functionaries have been implicated, as is indicated by studies from Uganda, Botswana and Tanzania (de Bruyn, 1992; Hartwig, 1991). In this punitive climate, women's symptoms and experience of HIV infection may be neglected, or they may be subjected to excessive discipline and control through routine screening at ante-natal clinics (often without consent) or, if HIV positive and pregnant, be pressured to undergo abortions.

Women themselves blame the sexual double standard. In Uganda, Barnett and Blaikie (1992: 106) were told: 'Women fear what their husbands may bring home', and: 'Women are innocent. They are dying for nothing' (1992: 106). In Tanzania, an AIDS researcher was repeatedly asked by women: 'What can we do about our husbands?' (Hartwig, 1991: 173).

The empowerment of women is an insistent theme in the literature on gender and AIDS in Africa. The perceived vulnerability of women to infection is regarded as variously linked to their economic dependency on men, their lack of control over sexual relations, and their need to conceive to gain social recognition. Empowerment is seen as a means whereby women can withstand male pressure and thereby counter their economic and normative lack of power. It is sometimes argued that when women empower themselves as a strategy for protection against AIDS, this can provide a basis for 'furthering women's emancipation' more generally (deBruyn, 1992: 259).

The means to empowerment has been seen to lie in harnessing the energies embodied in women's informal organizations to the task of devising collective strategies for protection. Ulin (1992: 64) argues that throughout much of Africa, 'rural women have always found strength in collective organizations, organizing themselves around specific needs and activities, using kinship ties, neighbourhood groups, and other informal networks to accomplish their aims'. This strength has not been fully recognized or utilized by policy makers in respect of AIDS campaigns, yet such informal associations may be a 'powerful vehicle for normative change' to the extent that they mobilize women's collective perceptions of their ability to respond to the AIDS threat (Ulin, 1992: 67).

The struggle against AIDS may actually be one of the most propitious for the empowerment of women. Given that HIV/AIDS is no respecter of class, age, ethnic or national boundaries, the fear it induces is experienced by all who are sexually active. Differences between women which may loom large in other contexts, dividing one from another, may be rendered insignificant when set against the threat of AIDS. And whilst people with AIDS may be stigmatized, any woman could be invisibly infected by HIV. As Noerine Kaleeba, founder of TASO in Uganda, says in her courageous book: 'I chose to conduct myself as if I was infected ... AIDS affects a cross section of people. AIDS affects *you and me*' (our italics; Kaleeba,1991: 42, 80).

There are beginning to be many instances of women coming together in the struggle to protect themselves against HIV/AIDS in Africa. In some areas, sex workers have been successful in rejecting clients who would not use condoms (an example from Nigeria is quoted in de Bruyn, 1992: 257; others from Mali and Kenya in Ulin, 1992: 67). In Nigeria, the success of the sex workers' stand was related to their active support for each other, as well as backing from hotel managers and older women sex workers. In Kenya, 'highly interactive community meetings' amongst prostitutes preceded high levels of commitment to use of condoms (Ulin, 1992: 67).

There are instances when women are able to call on 'community' support. Obbo (1993: 24) cites the case of a first wife who, because of her fear of AIDS, refused sexual relations with her husband and was backed up by neighbours when he tried to assert his conjugal 'rights'. The institution of polygamy worked to her favour here in that her husband was seen as having 'another venue for sexual enjoyment'. It more often works against women's need to protect themselves, as we illustrate below.

More organized approaches are also in evidence. At one level is the Society of Women and AIDS in Africa (SWAA) with its branches in many countries, which explicitly addresses itself to women's concerns while seeing campaigns to win over men as being vital to its success. At another level are local associations, such as TASO (The AIDS Support Organization) in Uganda, or WAMATA (Walio Katika Mapambano na AIDS Tanzania) in Tanzania, which whilst not addressing themselves exclusively to women, have found gender relations to be a key factor. 'We started in June 1989 with five families, as a voluntary, non-sectarian, non-governmental grass-roots organisa- tion, based on the spirit of solidarity, love and hope, to provide medical and nursing care, counselling, and to some extent material assistance to people living with HIV/AIDS. *All the gender issues we had never tackled came up at once'* (our italics; Waijage, 1993: 254).

These initiatives are not without their problems. SWAA has drawn fire from those who see its stance on male power as equivocal, demonstrated by a 'fear to address the African male directly with the consequences of his unrestrained and unchallenged dominance of the African woman' (Ankrah, 1991: 971). If projects are initiated by poor and illiterate women they may lack the knowledge of how to get funding (*AIDS Analysis Africa*, 1(4), 1991: 12); conversely, AIDS work can be an 'opportunity' for those who are already well-endowed to enhance their economic and social position: a form of con-sultancy entrepreneurialism that has been noted in many parts of the world (see, for example, Mbilinyi, 1987). Where projects represent genuine and spontaneous grassroots concern they can be too challenging to those in power; conversely, they may be taken up so enthusiastically that they collapse under the weight of responsibility and are discredited (Townsend, 1993). Groups organized by women may find themselves locked into the conven-tional female role of supporting men and families more than protecting themselves. And this voluntary work can be seen by the state as a substitute for public provision when structural adjustment policies bite deep.

One of the key contradictions in empowering women in the struggle against AIDS is that a new assertiveness of women may alienate men. This suggests the importance of an approach intrinsically sensitive to gender relations and the necessity of addressing the circumstances of both men and women.

Bringing Men on Board

Radical feminism identified men as 'the main enemy'. In the context of the struggle against HIV/AIDS in Africa, Christine Obbo (1993) has asserted that: 'Men are the Solution'. What is evident in the literature on Africa, given that the predominant mode of transmission of the AIDS virus is through heterosexual sex, is that women cannot protect themselves without a corre-sponding change in male behaviour and response. Herein lies a paradox, for the power of men over women must be challenged at the same time as men must be won over to more mutuality in sexual relations. Waijage's (1993) earlier comment: 'all the gender issues we had never tackled came up at once', bears testimony to this difficulty.

Ulin (1992: 64) comments that though the solidarity of African women may be their greatest source of strength in combatting and coping with AIDS, they cannot cope alone. 'They must be empowered to share the responsibility with men, participating equally in personal and community strategies to block transmissions of the virus.' Because issues of sexuality and sexual norms are so deeply embedded in complex socio-cultural settings, and because of the importance of fertility to women's status, women's knowledge and even women's action on its own cannot ensure protection. As Carovano notes (1991: 49): 'To provide women exclusively with HIV protection methods that contradict most societies' fertility norms is to provide many women with no options at all.' To choose childlessness is not an option for women in Africa, and in order to have children women must engage in 'unprotected sex', putting themselves at risk. Obbo's (1993: 240) bleak report on Uganda is telling: 'Celibacy is an acceptable option for widows who are grateful to be alive and uninfected and do not want to tempt fate – because the next time they may not escape AIDS.'

This does not mean that the issue of the potentially fatal consequences of cultural norms can be avoided. Noerine Kaleeba reported that her husband's desire for a son led him to enter into an affair with another woman who may have infected him, but that she knew of this and accepted it: 'polygamy was something we had all grown up with' (Kaleeba, 1991: 9). Msaky (1992: 10) reports that 'traditionally', 'for a man to have multiple sexual partners used to be a sign of wealth, of which he was proud' (see also Nzioka, 1994). Now polygamy, along with the sexual exploitation by older men of young girls (the 'sugar daddy' phenomenon) and the sexual double standard are all in question, and these are issues of gender politics which also raise issues of economic power. When women question men's time-honoured rights over them they are often subject to violence, abuse and the withdrawal of livelihood (a 'male backlash' as the Tanzania Gender Networking Programme describes it), and the state may provide a legal and ideological framework for this (Ampofu, 1993; Msaky, 1992; Phillips, 1994; TGNP, 1993).

In the context of the AIDS epidemic, men may divorce wives who test HIV positive, and the wives of men with AIDS are often disinherited. A poignant personal example is related by Schoepf (1993: 254):

> In 1988 Mbeya became aware that her husband was sick and not getting any better. She began to suspect that it might be AIDS, and told him she wanted to use condoms. Her husband refused. So she said they should stop sexual relations. Her husband's family was outraged and he refused this too. They threatened to throw her out and keep her youngest daughter. Mbeya acquiesced. Following her husband's death, her in-laws accused her of infecting her husband.

Mbeya's husband was rich, but all his property, including their house, was then taken by his relatives. As Schoepf (1993: 254) concludes: 'Social structure limits the ability of women to become independent actors exercising social agency'.

It is against, but also in recognition of, this threatening reality that women must bring men on board in the fight against HIV/AIDS. If at one level this means paying closer attention to men's behaviour and attitudes (McGrath *et al.*, 1993), at another it means ensuring men's appreciation of the fact that their own survival, as well as that of their partners and children, is intimately bound up with the way in which sexual relations are structured. It may be of strategic importance to legitimate changes sought as being of ultimate benefit to both men and women, with gains in health being shown to outweigh any accompanying losses to men's sexual domination over women.

Yet it is also appreciated that this is not the end of the matter. Men may have good reason to fear that the empowerment of women in respect of sexuality and sexual relations could have an impact on other aspects of gendered (power) relations.[6] Indeed, it might presage greater autonomy for women generally and perhaps a realization of strategic gender needs. Understandably then, men are torn between their desire for life and the loss of their control over women. But as one young man reported to Obbo (1993: 243): 'Men infect young girls and their wives. Men must change their behaviours or else we face extinction.'

A recognition of this stark reality in some areas of Africa is highlighted by developments that promote more gender equity. The routes may be various – the importation of protective technology (the female condom), which is under women's control; the endorsement of condom use by at least one head of state (President Museveni in Uganda: Obbo 1993: 242); the public challenging of existing sexual practices or norms of sexuality by the state or by women's organizations; and the very rise of grassroots associations expressing women's collective strength and providing support to individual women in relations with their partners.

Methodological Issues

Any work in the field of HIV/AIDS that affirms the value (indeed necessity) of empowerment should be self-consciously aware of the way in which methods of research or of project implementation facilitate or inhibit empowerment. A research initiative that is exclusively oriented towards interviewing individual women (or individual men) about their sexual behaviour may generate useful knowledge that could be applied in planning personal strategies of protection. It may even heighten individual consciousness of how the exercise of power in sexual relations operates, or of the obstacles to individual attempts to bring about change. It may empower in the sense of 'enlightening'. But it cannot of itself ensure that change will be broad or long lasting (Holland *et al.*, 1992).

A contrasting method that is being used increasingly in HIV/AIDS research in Africa bears directly on the way in which sexuality and norms of sexual relations, as well as being privately exercised, are also the subject of public knowledge. This is the 'focus group', involving guided group discussion around a particular topic (Brown *et al.*, 1993; Hunter, 1990; Irwin *et al.*, 1991; Konde-Lule *et al.*, 1993; Nabaitu *et al.*, 1992). It has particular merit in linking the generation of research 'data' with collective consciousness raising and holds the potential for linking both to the generation of strategies of protection. In practice, focus groups have been organized on various lines of difference – e.g. groups of grandparents, of young women, of young men, etc.– but they could be a precursor to wider debate that cuts across such social categories of difference.

The focus group implies a degree of collective participation in the phase of data collection. It can also be used at other stages of an avowedly participatory approach – not just involving research but also interventions. Individualistic interventions are as limited in their value as are individually-focused research methodologies.

Health education approaches that aim to inform, assuming that information delivered to individuals is sufficient in itself and ignoring the social relations of power in which the information must be put into use, have been shown to be less than effective. In Kenya, 94 women revealed to be HIV positive were individually counselled at Pumwani Maternity Hospital in Nairobi to use condoms and inform their spouses. They were also informed of the risks of pregnancy-related transmission. At a follow-up one year later, only 24 could be traced. Their use of condoms or of oral contraceptives was low, only nine had informed their partners and most 'expressed the desire to have even more babies to increase the number of uninfected children' (Temmerman *et al.*, 1993: 105).

Compare the success of a more collective approach. In Zaire, a report on work with women sex-workers (15) and with churchwomen (60) using methods of collective empowerment through active learning techniques, which addressed women's structural dependency on men and their capacity to support each other in protecting themselves, showed that after three months all the sex-workers but one were using condoms, but that after eight months their usage had declined following claims by clients that condoms were ineffective. After two of the women died of AIDS all the rest began to use condoms. One third of the churchwomen reported having been able to persuade their husbands, in principle, to use condoms (Schoepf *et al.*, 1993: 219–24).

A research methodology which is self-consciously based on collective participation and which facilitates collective action is more than an important accompaniment to methodologies using conventional techniques. It is essential in this field.

Conclusions

In this chapter we have traced an intellectual history transversing several fields of theory and practice. We have examined the way in which the concept of empowerment, and the related concept of power, have been used in a variety of literatures, all of which bear on strategies for combatting the threat of HIV/AIDS in Africa. In making a critical assessment of this literature, we have come to a range of conclusions. What struck us at first was that the adoption of empowerment as a strategy in the AIDS field (by gay activists in Europe and America and by self-help and women's groups in Africa) seemed to echo the utilization of empowerment as a strategic way of addressing the problems of disadvantage in the developing world by agencies working in the development field. In our view, the eagerness with which 'empowerment' has been seized upon by external agencies as a solution to the ills of poverty, ill health, racism or sexism betrayed a failure to confront power relations in which such agencies may themselves be implicated, and displaced responsibility for disadvantage onto the shoulders of those who are its victims.

Conversely, in the politics of new-wave feminism, empowerment had a proven history of success: new-wave feminism did change (if not totally transform) the world, and its diverse theories were based on an analysis of gendered power. More recently, feminism, in its engagement with current debates within the social sciences around the challenge of poststructuralism and postmodernism, has deconstructed the concept and reality of 'power', and questioned the assumption that it is structurally based. A postmodernist critique has also been one of the factors leading to an 'impasse' in development theory. From our perspective (assessing strategies to stem the spread of AIDS, especially for women), these theoretical developments, while they offer novel lines of investigation (discourses of sexuality/power), represent a backward step, making it difficult to confront power in its various forms.

Looking again at the literature on HIV/AIDS activism, we concluded that empowerment can be a forceful and effective means to people changing their behaviour, but it is so only to the extent that it moves beyond individualistic 'enlightenment' formulas and embraces a collective form. The danger of the former is that 'knowledge' wilts before power in its various guises; but there are also inherent difficulties in the latter, given that the essentially privatized nature of sexual encounters (the lonely moment of the sexual embrace) eludes collective intervention and support. Empowerment initiatives have to recognize existing relations of economic and political power in which women are enmeshed, as well as acknowledging the various subversive and confrontational ways in which women have already been able to challenge them. It is this recognition and acknowledgement that can provide a basis for action in the arena of life and death struggles defined by AIDS.

Research aimed at facilitating (as opposed to simply observing and analysing) empowerment should utilize reflexive methodologies capable of fostering and releasing collective potentiality. Participatory methods might be useful in this respect, but not sufficient unless participation is extended from the research process towards locally generated initiatives to confront and transform behaviour and to challenge existing gender relations.

Assessing the effectiveness of collective action in this field throws up all the issues which sociologists long ago identified from a variety of perspectives, and which still need to be confronted: issues of agency versus structure, the links between micro-level politics and state power, the political economy of resistance, interests groups and their competitive political claims, institutional-ization, bureaucracy and the routinization of charisma.

Finally, it is clear that a strictly medical discourse is inadequate to deal with a problem embedded (literally) in human relations, and that a halt to epidemic trends requires these to change – hence the message of 'safer sex'. On one level this is clearly a message of repression and discipline (a 'discourse' of sexuality of the kind that Foucault revealed) delivered in élitist fashion by 'experts' to the 'ignorant'. But there is scope for exploring the contradictions here – for safer sex is also a formula for life, for mutual respect and for human emancipation. If it is to be achieved, in a gender-aware fashion, feminists cannot afford to abandon the 'emancipatory project', however tainted this may be perceived to be by Enlightenment thinking; it must operate with a vision tempered by recognition of the complexity of its achievement.

Acknowledgement

Earlier versions of this paper were presented at the annual conference of the British Sociological Association, Preston, 1994, and at the Overseas Develop-ment Group's conference on Gender Research and Development: Looking Forward to Beijing, Norwich, 1994. We are grateful for helpful criticisms received from participants.

Notes

1   An ESRC funded research project on Gender Relations as a Key Aspect in the Fight Against HIV/AIDS in Tanzania and Zambia (ESRC Ref. R000 23 5221).

2   Barrett implies that it is impossible, and that it is this which has led some to abandon structuralist approaches (1991: 73–4).

3   In an interview in 1983, Foucault remarked 'I must confess that I am much more interested in problems about techniques of the self ... than sex ... sex is boring'

(in Rabinow, 1984: 340).

4   Maximum condoms have swept the market, selling 4.5 million in 1993. USAID is cooperating in this endeavour with the Pharmaceutical Society of Zambia, a parastatal which distributes the brand. *Weekly Post,* Zambia, 21 January 1994/23 November 1993.

5   The seemingly innocuous enterprise of teaching women to read and write has sometimes sown the seeds of rebellion against gender inequities. A recent report described how women in India campaigned against the sale of government liquor because the men who buy it squander family resources and beat their wives and children. The protest, which cut across caste and class lines, began with poor illiterate village women in Andra Pradesh discussing a story produced for a literacy campaign. 'The village women began attacking liquor shops, pouring the alcohol into the streets and shaving the heads of men found drunk there … they seized drunken patrons, wrapped skirts around them and paraded them on donkeys' (*Guardian,* 28 December 1993).

6   Kate Young (1993: 159) makes a related and broader point in reference to empowerment of women necessarily entailing a loss of men's power: 'empowerment is not just about women acquiring something, but about those holding power relinquishing it.'

References

AMPOFU, A.A. (1993) 'Controlling and punishing women: violence against Ghanaian women', *Review of African Political Economy,* **56**, 102–111.

ANKRAH, M. (1991) 'AIDS and the social side of health', *Social Science and Medicine,* **32**(9), 967–80.

BARRETT, T. and BLAIKIE, P. (1992) *AIDS in Africa: Its Present and Future Impact,* Belhaven Press.

BARRETT, M. (1980) *Women's Oppression Today,* London: Verso.

BARRETT, M. (1987) 'The concept of "Difference"', *Feminist Review,* **26**, 29–41.

BARRETT, M. (1991) *The Politics of Truth,* Cambridge: Polity Press.

BARRETT, M. and PHILLIPS, A. (1992) *Destabilising Theory: Contemporary Feminist Debates,* Cambridge: Polity Press.

BASSETT, M. and MHLOYI, M. (1991) 'Women and AIDS in Zimbabwe: the making of an epidemic', *International Journal of Health Services,* **21**(1), 143–56.

BORDO, S. (1993) 'Feminism, Foucault and the politics of the body', in RAMAZANOGLU, C. (Ed.) *Up Against Foucault: Explorations of Some Tensions between Foucault and Feminism,* London: Routledge.

BROWN, J.E., AYOWA, O.B. and BROWN, C. (1993) 'Dry and tight: sexual practices and potential AIDS risk in Zaire', *Social Science and Medicine,* **37**(8), 989–94.

BUJRA, J. (1993) 'Power and empowerment; a tale of two Tanzanian servants', *Review of African Political Economy,* **56**, 68–78.

CAROVANO, K. (1991) 'More than mothers and whores: Redefining the AIDS prevention needs of women', *International Journal of Health Services,* **21**(1), 429–39.

CHAMBERS, R. (1992) 'Methods for analysis by farmers: the professional challenge', paper presented to the Association for Farming Systems Research/Extensions 1991–2 Symposium, Michigan State University.

COOTE, A. and CAMPBELL, B. (1987) *Sweet Freedom*, Oxford: Basil Blackwell.

DAVIS, K., LEIJENAAR, M. and OLDERSMA, J. (Eds) (1991) *The Gender of Power*, London: Sage.

DE BRUYN, M. (1992) 'Women and AIDS in developing countries', *Social Science and Medicine*, **34**(3), 249–62.

DELPHY, C. (1980) 'A materialist feminism is possible', *Feminist Review*, **4**, 79–105.

DELSING, R. (1991) 'Sovereign and disciplinary power: a Foucauldian analysis of the Chilean women's movement', in DAVIS, K., LEIJENAAR, M. and OLDERSMA, J. (Eds) *The Gender of Power*, London: Sage.

EDWARDS, M. (1993) 'How relevant is development studies?', in SCHUURMAN, F.J. (Ed.) *Beyond the Impasse: New Directions in Development Theory*, London: Zed Press.

FERNANDES, W. and TANDON, R. (1981) 'Social research for social Action: an introduction', in FERNANDES, W. and TANDON, R. (Eds) *Participatory Research and Evaluation: Experiments in Research as a Process of Liberation*, New Delhi: Indian Social Institute.

FIRESTONE, S. (1970) *The Dialectic of Sex*, New York: Wm. Morrow and Company.

FOUCAULT, M. (1980A) 'THE EYE OF POWER', IN GORDON, C. (Ed.) *Power/Knowledge*, New York, Harvester Wheatsheaf.

FOUCAULT, M. (1980B) 'POWER AND STRATEGIES', IN GORDON, C. (Ed.) *Power/Knowledge*, New York, Harvester Wheatsheaf.

FOUCAULT, M. (1980C) 'TRUTH AND POWER', IN GORDON, C. (Ed.) *Power/Knowledge*, New York, Harvester Wheatsheaf.

FOUCAULT, M. (1979) *Discipline and Punish*, New York: Vintage.

FOUCAUL, M. (1984) *The History of Sexuality*, vol 1, Harmondsworth: Penguin.

FREEMAN, J. (1971) 'The tyranny of structurelessness', *The Second Wave*, **2** 1.

FREIDAN, B. (1963) *The Feminine Mystique*. New York: Dell.

FRIEDMANN, J. (1992) *Empowerment: The politics of alternative development*, Oxford: Blackwell.

GATENS, M. (1992) 'Power, bodies and difference', in BARRETT, M. and PHILLIPS, A. (Eds), *Destabilising Theory: Contemporary Feminist Debates*, Cambridge: Polity Press.

HARTWIG, K. (1991) 'The politics of AIDS in Tanzania: Gender perceptions and the challenges for educational strategies', unpublished MA thesis, Clark University, Massachussets, USA.

HOLLAND, J., RAMAZANOGLU, C. and SCOTT, S. (1990) 'AIDS: From panic stations to power relations: sociological perspectives and problems' *Sociology*, **24**, 3.

HOLLAND, J., RAMAZANOGLU, C., SCOTT, S., SHARPE, S. and THOMSON (1992) 'Risk, power and the possibility of pleasure: young women and safer sex', *AIDS Care*, **4**, 3.

HUNTER, S. (1990) 'Orphans as a window on the AIDS epidemic in sub-saharan Africa: initial results and implications of a study in Uganda', *Social Science and Medicine*, **31**(6), 681–90.

IRWIN, K., BERTRAND, J., MILANDUMBA, N., *et al.*, (1991) 'Knowledge, attitudes and beliefs about HIV infection and AIDS among factory workers and their wives, Kinshasa, Zaire', *Social Science and Medicine*, **32**(8), 917–30.

KALEEBA, N. (1991) *We Miss You All: AIDS in the Family*, Harare: Zimbabwe, Women and AIDS Support Network.

KAIJAGE, T. (1993) 'WAMATA: People striving to control the spread of AIDS, Tanzania', in BERER, M. and RAY, S. *Women and HIV/AIDS: An International Resource Book*, London: Pandora.

KIPPAX, S. (1992) 'The importance of gay community in the prevention of HIV transmission', in AGGLETON, P., DAVIES, P. and HART, G. (Eds) *AIDS: Rights, Risk and Reason*, London: Falmer Press.

KITZINGER, J. and MILLER, J. (1991) 'In black and white: A preliminary report on the role of the media in audience understandings of "African AIDS"', paper presented to the Fifth conference on Social Aspects of AIDS, South Bank Polytechnic, 23 March.

KONDE-LULE, J.K., MUSAGARA, M. and MUSGRAVE, M. (1993) 'Focus group interviews about AIDS in Rakai District of Uganda' *Social Science and Medicine*, **37**(5), 679–84.

LERNER, B. (1964) *The Passing of Traditional Society*, New York: The Free Press.

LONG, N. (1990) 'From paradigm lost to paradigm regained? The case for an actor-oriented sociology of development', *European Review of Latin American and Caribbean Studies*, **49**, 3–24.

LONG, N. and VILLAREAL, M. (1993) 'Exploring development interfaces: from the transfer of knowledge to the transformation of meaning', in SCHUURMAN, F. (Ed.) *Beyond the Impasse: New Directions in Development Theory*, London: Zed Books.

LONGWE, S.H. (1991) 'Gender awareness: the missing element in the Third World development project', in WALLACE, T. (Ed.) *Changing Perceptions: Writings on Gender and Development*, Oxford: Oxfam.

LOVIBOND, S. (1990) 'Feminism and postmodernism', in BOYNE, R. and RATTANSI, A. (Eds), *Postmodernism and Society*, Basingstoke: Macmillan.

MACKINTOSH, M. (1989) *Gender, Class and Rural Transition*, London: Zed Press.

MACLURE, R. and BASSEY, M. (1991) 'Participatory action research in Togo: An enquiry into maize storage systems', in FOOTE WHYTE, W. (Ed.) *Participatory Action Research*, London: Sage.

MBILINYI, M. (1987) '"Women in Development" Ideology and the Marketplace', in MINER, V. and LONGINO, S. (Eds) *Competition: A Feminist Taboo?* New York: The Feminist Press.

McGRATH, J.W., Rwabukwali, C., Schumann, D., *et al.* (1993) 'Anthropology and AIDS: the cultural context of sexual risk behaviour amongst urban Baganda women in Kampala, Uganda', *Social Science and Medicine*, **36**(4), 429–39.

McKEVITT, C. (1993) 'Solidarity, empowerment, AIDS and anthropology', paper given at the British Association for Anthropology in Policy and Practice, conference on HIV and AIDS in Europe: The Challenge for Anthropology, London: South Bank University, 19–20 February.

McNEIL, M. (1993) 'Dancing with Foucault: feminism and power-knowledge', in RAMAZANOGLU, C. (Ed.), *Up Against Foucault: Explorations of Some Tensions between Foucault and Feminism*, London: Routledge.

MOHANTY, C. (1992) 'Feminist encounters: locating the politics of experience', in BARRETT, M. and PHILLIPS, A. (Eds) *Destabilising Theory: Contemporary Feminist Debates*, Cambridge: Polity Press.

MOLYNEUX, M. (1985) 'Mobilisation without emancipation? Women's interests, state and revolution in Nicaragua', *Feminist Studies*, **11**(2), 27–254.

MOSER, C. (1993) *Gender Planning and Development: Theory, Practice, Training*, London: Routledge.

Msaky, H.I. (1992) 'Women, AIDS and sexual violence in Africa', *Vena Journal*, **4**, 2.

Nabaitu, J., Kajura, E., Seeley, J. and Mulder, D. (1992) 'Community perceptions of determinants of sexual behaviour in rural Uganda', paper given at the Eighth International Conference on AIDS, Amsterdam.

Obbo, C. (1993) 'HIV transmission: men are the solution', in James, S. and Busia, A. (Eds) *Theorising Black Feminisms*, London: Routledge.

Ojanuga, D.N. and Gilbert, C. (1992) 'Women's access to health care in developing countries', *Social Science and Medicine*, **35**(4), 613–7.

Opie, A. (1992) 'Qualitative research: Appropriation of the "Other" and empowerment.', *Feminist Review*, **40**, 52–69.

Pearson, R. (1993) 'Different discourses: Women in development; Gender analysis in development and feminism', paper presented to the Conference of Socialist Economists, Leeds.

Phillips, O. (1994) 'Censuring sexuality and gender in Zimbabawe: a look at some moral panics', paper presented to the British Sociological Association Annual conference, Preston.

Pitts, M. and Jackson, H. (1993) 'Press coverage of AIDS in Zimbabwe: A five year review', *AIDS Care*, **5**, 2.

Pringle, R. and Watson, S. (1992) ' "Women's interests" and the post-structuralist state', in Barrett, M. and Phillips, A. (Eds) *Destabilising Theory: Contemporary Feminist Debates*, Cambridge: Polity Press.

Rabinow, P. (Ed.) (1984) *The Foucault Reader*, Harmondsworth: Penguin.

Rahnemar, R. (1992) 'Participation', in Sachs, W. (Ed.) *The Development Dictionary*, London: Zed Books.

Ramazanoglu, C. (1993) *Up Against Foucault: Explorations of Some Tensions between Foucault and Feminism*, London: Routledge.

Ramazanoglu, C. and Holland, J. (1993) 'Women's sexuality and men's appropriation of desire', in Ramazanoglu, C. (Ed.) *Up Against Foucault: Explorations of Some Tensions between Foucault and Feminism*, London: Routledge.

Salmen, L. (1987) *Listen to the People: Participant Observer Evaluation of Development Projects*, New York: Oxford University Press for the World Bank.

Schoepf, B. (1991) 'Ethical, methodological and political issues of AIDS research in central Africa', *Social Science and Medicine*, **33**(7), 749–63.

Shoepf, B. (1993) 'Women at risk: case studies from Zaire', in Berer, M. and Ray, S. *Women and HIV/AIDS: An International Resource Book*, London: Pandora.

Schoepf, B., Engundu, W., Rukarangira, W.N., Ntsomo, P. and Schoepf, C. (1991) 'Gender, power and risk of AIDS in Zaire', in Turshen, M. (Ed.) *Women and Health in Africa*, Trenton, NJ: Africa World Press.

Schoepf, B. with Engundu, W., Wenkeru, R., Nlsomo, P. and Schoepf, C. (1993) 'Empowerment through "risk reduction workshops"', in Berer, M. and Ray, S. *Women and HIV/AIDS: An International Resource Book*, London: Pandora, 219–224.

Schuurman, F. (1993) *Beyond the Impasse: New Directions in Development Theory*, London: Zed Books.

Seeley, J., Kengeya-Kayondo, J. and Maider, D. (1992) 'Community-based HIV/AIDS research – whither community participation? Unsolved problems in a research programme in rural Uganda', *Social Science and Medicine*, **34**(10), 1089–95.

Seidel, G. (1993) 'The competing discourses of HIV/AIDS in Sub-Saharan Africa:

Discourses of rights and empowerment vs discourses of control and exclusion', *Social Science and Medicine*, **36**(3), 175–94.

SSALI, A., BARTON, T., KATONGLE, G. and SEELEY, J. (1992) 'Exploring sexual terminology in a vernacular in rural Uganda: lessons for health education', paper presented to the VIII International conference on AIDS, Amsterdam.

TANZANIA GENDER NETWORKING PROGRAMME (TGNP) (1993) *Gender Profile of Tanzania*, Dar es Salaam, Tanzania: TGNP.

TEMMERMAN, M., MOSES, S., KARAGU, D., FUSALLAH, S., AMOLA, I. and PIOT, P. (1993) 'Post-partum counselling of HIV infected women and their subsequent repro-ductive behaviour', in BERER, M. and RAY, S. (Eds) *Women and HIV/AIDS: An International Resource Book*, London: Pandora.

TOWNSEND, J. (1993) 'Gender studies: whose agenda?', in SCHUURMAN, F.J. (Ed.) *Beyond the Impasse: New Directions in Development Studies*, London: Zed Books.

ULIN, P. (1992) 'African women and AIDS: negotiating behavioural change', *Social Science and Medicine*, **34**(1), 63–73.

WAIJAGE, T. (1993) 'WAMATA: People striving to control the spread of AIDS, Tanzania', in BERER, M. and RAY, S. *Women and HIV/AIDS: An International Resource Book*, London: Pandora.

WINSBURY R. (1992) 'AIDS and the multi-nationals: corporate policy and practice towards HIV in Africa', *AIDS Analysis Africa*, **2**(6), 7.

WORLD BANK (1990) *World Development Report: Investing in Health*, Washington.

YOUNG, K. (1993) *Planning Development with Women: Making a World of Difference*, London: Macmillan.

Notes on Contributors

Philippe Adam is a sociologist attached to the CERMES in Paris. He is working on a study of gay male adaptation to the AIDS epidemic as well as studying French AIDS activism. He is co-author (with Claudine Herzlich) of *Sociologie de la maladie et de la médicine* (Nathan Université, Collection Sociologie, 1994).

Derek Adam-Smith is a senior lecturer in Industrial Relations at the University of Portsmouth Business School where, with David Goss, he founded the Centre for AIDS and Employment Research. He has written widely on the subject of HIV/AIDS and employment, including (with David Goss) *Organising AIDS: Workplace and Organisational Responses to the HIV/AIDS Epidemic* (Taylor & Francis, 1995).

Peter Aggleton is Professor in Education, and co-director of the Health and Education Research Unit at the Institute of Education, University of London. He has worked internationally in HIV/AIDS health promotion, and is currently coordinating a major programme of social and behavioural research for the World Health Organisation's Global Programme on AIDS. His publications include *Deviance* (Tavistock, 1987); *Health* (Routledge, 1990); *AIDS: Rights, Risk and Reason* (Ed. with Peter Davies and Graham Hart, Taylor & Francis, 1992); *AIDS: Facing the Second Decade* (Ed. with Peter Davies and Graham Hart, Taylor & Francis, 1993) and *AIDS: Foundations for the Future* (Ed. with Peter Davies and Graham Hart, Taylor & Francis, 1994).

Dennis Altman is Professor in Politics at La Trobe University, Melbourne. He is the author of eight books, including *Power and Community: Organisational and Cultural Responses to AIDS* (Taylor & Francis, 1994), *AIDS and New Puritanism* (Pluto, 1986), and *Homosexual: Oppression and Liberation* (Penguin, 1972, new edition New York University Press, 1993). His first novel, *The Comfort of Men*, was published by Heinemann in 1993. He is a member of the Global AIDS

AIDS Policy Coalition and of the committee of the International Council of AIDS Service Organizations, and has served on a variety of AIDS advisory bodies in Australia.

Carolyn Baylies is a senior lecturer in Sociology at the University of Leeds. She has carried out research in Zambia on electoral politics, class formation and the state and democratization, and has also published work on indigenous enterprise, gender and health.

Mary Boulton is Senior Lecturer in Sociology as Applied to Medicine at St Mary's Hospital Medical School (Imperial College), University of London. She has worked extensively investigating the factors contributing to the sexual behaviour of gay and bisexual men in relation to HIV/AIDS and is currently involved in research on the experience of families with HIV-infected children and on the social aspects of genetic screening. She is editor of *Challenge and Innovation: Methodological Advances in Social Research on HIV/AIDS* (Taylor & Francis,1994).

Janet Bujra is presently a senior lecturer in the Department of Peace Studies, at the University of Bradford. She has carried out research in Tanzania and Kenya on domestic service, prostitution, labour migration, housing and political action, and has also published work on gender, class, ethnicity and economic development.

Stephen Clift is Reader in Health Education in the Centre for Health Education and Research, Canterbury Christchurch College, Canterbury. He has worked in the area of HIV/AIDS education and young people since 1986 and has produced several resources to support HIV/AIDS and sex education with young people. These include *HIV/AIDS and Sex: Information for Young People* (AVERT, 1994, 3rd edition) and *Condoms, Pills and Other Useful things* (AVERT, 1994). He is editor (with Stephen Page) of *Health and the International Tourist*, (Routledge, 1995), and (with Peter Grabowski) *Tourism and Health: Risks, Research and Responses* (Cassell, forthcoming).

June Crawford is a senior lecturer in the School of Behavioural Sciences at Macquarie University, Australia, where she has been involved in HIV/AIDS research since 1987. Her recent publications have appeared in the *Australian Journal of Psychology* and *The National Centre for Epidemiology and Population Health Working Papers Series*. She is also co-author of *Emotion and Gender: Constructing Meaning from Memory* (Sage, 1992).

Peter Davies is Director of Research in the School of Health Studies at the University of Portsmouth. He is a Principal Investigator of SIGMA Research and author of *Key Texts in Multidimensional Scaling* (Heinemann, 1982); *Images of Social Stratification* (Sage, 1985); and co-author (with Ford Hickson, Peter Weatherburn and Andrew Hunt) of *Sex, Gay Men and AIDS* (Taylor & Francis, 1993). He is editor (with Peter Aggleton and Graham Hart) of *AIDS: Responses, Interventions and Care* (Taylor & Francis, 1991); *AIDS: Risk, Rights and Reason* (Taylor & Francis, 1992); *AIDS: Facing the Second Decade* (Taylor & Francis, 1993); and *AIDS: Foundations for the Future* (Taylor & Francis, 1994).

Katie Deverell is the Senior Research Officer for The HIV Project, London. She is also registered for a part-time PhD at Keele University, researching the construction of sexual boundaries in HIV-related outreach work. Her most recent publications include (with Alan Prout) *MESMAC Working with Diversity – Building Communities, Evaluating the MESMAC Project* (London, HEA, 1995) and (with Michael Rooney) *Using Sexually Explicit Materials for Safer Sex Work with Gay Men* (London, The HIV Project, 1994).

Ana Filgueiras is with the Hand-in-Hand Network in Rio de Janeiro, Brazil.

Deirdre Fullerton is a research fellow in the Social Science Research Unit at the Institute of Education, University of London. Her research interests include the design, development and evaluation of health education interventions.

Philip Gatter is Senior Research Fellow in Anthropology in the Social Sciences Research Centre, South Bank University, London. He has worked on the evaluation of HIV/AIDS social care services, and is currently writing a book on 'Identity, Sexuality, and AIDS' (Cassell, forthcoming). His other publications in this field have appeared in *AIDS Care, Social Science and Medicine* and *AIDS: Facing the Second Decade* (Taylor & Francis, 1993).

David Goss is Professor of Organisational Behaviour at the University of Portsmouth Business School where, with Derek Adam-Smith, he founded the Centre for AIDS and Employment Research. He has written widely on the subject of HIV/AIDS and employment, including (with Derek Adam-Smith) *Organising AIDS: Workplace and Organisational Responses to the HIV/AIDS Epidemic* (Taylor & Francis, 1995).

Gill Green is a research lecturer in the Department of Sociology at the University of Essex. She is working on a follow-up study of a sample of men and women with HIV in Scotland, which focuses on the psychosocial impact of an HIV-positive diagnosis and styles of stigma management. She is also interested in cross-cultural comparisons and women's sexual health.

Graham Hart is Assistant Director of the MRC Medical Sociology Unit,

University of Glasgow, where he directs a programme of research on Sexual and Reproductive Health. He has undertaken studies of risk in gay men, injecting drug users and sex workers, and published widely in the HIV/AIDS field. He is co-editor of the journal *AIDS Care*, and General Editor of the forthcoming series of books *Health, Risk and Society* (UCL Press).

Janet Holland is Lecturer in Education at the Open University and Senior Research Lecturer in the Social Science Research Unit at the Institute of Education, University of London. Her general research interests are in the area of gender, youth and class. She has undertaken research into young women's sexuality with the Women, Risk and AIDS Project.

Susan Kippax is Associate Professor in the School of Behavioural Sciences at Macquarie University, Australia. She has been involved in many aspects of HIV/AIDS research since 1986, and since 1990 has been the deputy director of the Australian National Centre in HIV Social Research. She is the author of numerous publications on the social aspects of AIDS, most recently in *AIDS*. She is also co-author of *Emotion and Gender: Constructing Meaning from Memory* (Sage, 1992).

Ann Oakley is Professor in Sociology and Social Policy and Director of the Social Science Research Unit at the Institute of Education, University of London. She has been researching the fields of gender, the family and health for 30 years. Her publications include *Becoming a Mother* (Martin Robertson, Oxford, 1979), *The Captured Womb: a history of medical care for pregnant women* (Blackwell, 1984), *Social Support and Motherhood* (Blackwell, 1992) and *Essays on Women, Medicine and Health* (Edinburgh University Press, 1993). Her recent work has been concerned with methodologies of evaluation and epistemologies of knowledge.

Alan Prout is a senior lecturer in the Department of Sociology and Social Anthropology at Keele University, and Course Director for the Centre for Medical Social Anthropology. Recent publications include a chapter in *Does it Work? Perspectives on the Evaluation of HIV/AIDS Health Promotion* (P. Aggleton *et al.* (Eds), Health Education Authority, 1992) and (with Katie Deverell) *Working with Diversity – Building Communities, Evaluating the MESMAC Project* (London, Health Education Authority, 1995).

Tim Rhodes is Research Fellow at The Centre for Research on Drugs and Health Behaviour, University of London. He is currently doing qualitative research into risk, HIV infection and sexual safety among opiate and stimulant users in London. Recent publications include *Risk, Intervention and Change: HIV Prevention and Drug Use* (London, Health Education Authority, 1994) and

AIDS, Drugs and Prevention: Perspectives on Individual and Community Action (London, Routledge, 1995).

Marie-Ange Schiltz is a researcher at the CNRS. Since 1985, she has participated in the annual study, of the lifestyles and adaptation to the AIDS epidemic of gay and bisexual French men. She has published in *Actes de la Recherche en Sciences Sociales, Anthropologie et Société*, and *AIDS Care*.

Catherine Waldby works at Murdoch University, Australia. She is the author of several publications on aspects of sexuality and AIDS, most recently in the journals *Sociology of Health and Illness, Social Semiotics* and *Southern Review*. She has recently completed a doctorate about AIDS biomedicine, sexual difference and the concept of the body politic.

John Wilkins is a public health specialist in the Department of Public Health, Merton, Sutton and Wandsworth Health Authority. He has been involved in HIV/AIDS health promotion since 1986 and in the commissioning of HIV/ AIDS care, treatment and prevention services since 1992. He has been associated with the Centre for Health Education and Research, Canterbury for the past five years.

Index